Moments
in the Death of a
Flesh Mechanic
...a healer's rebirth

Russ Reina

"Moments in the Death of a Flesh Mechanic…A Healer's Rebirth," by Russ Reina. ISBN 978-1-60264-565-3.

Library of Congress Control Number: 2010928584.

Published 2010 by Virtualbookworm.com Publishing Inc., P.O. Box 9949, College Station, TX 77842, US. ©2010, Russ Reina. All rights reserved. No part of this publication may be reproduced, stored in a retrieval system, or transmitted in any form or by any means, electronic, mechanical, recording or otherwise, without the prior written permission of Russ Reina.

Manufactured in the United States of America.

He was the biggest kid on any block.
"C'mon, let's play Tug-o-War," he said.
"Are you kidding?" I stammered.
"I can't pull you in to that stinky ol' ditch!"
"No worries," he replied,
"Just keep yourself from falling in!"

**To the pioneers,
and those whose hearts
got broken**

A NOTE ABOUT THE BOOK
(Ye Olde Disclaimer!)

The events described in this book took place during the earliest phases of a new way of delivering emergency medical care in the United States. Since then, therapies and interventions, drugs and delivery systems, protocols and procedures, and companies and institutions have all gone through quite a bit of evolution.

Some of the drugs and interventions I used in the field have gone out of favor, if not been discredited or banned from use altogether. Please keep in mind, twenty-five years from now many of the procedures in use today will have suffered the same fate!

This is not a manual of emergency care. It is a window into the interior life of a paramedic dealing the best he could with the systems he was part of, using the tools available to him under the circumstances of the times.

But, since we're on the subject…if I tell you a procedure I used worked, it worked. Maybe just for me; that, after all, is part of the Great Mystery!

I experienced everything written about in this book. Some identifying characteristics have been changed to protect saints, sinners and myself. I have created composite people and situations and manipulated time while remaining true to the key elements as they happened with each call. If you searched, you'd find enough verifiable details to let me slide on the illustrative embellishments I employed to serve better your understanding of the interior and exterior worlds I describe.

This is but one part of my life in the healing arts. For the big picture, go to http://www.firetender.org. Here I offer you a free resource to help you expand your capabilities in any healing art you practice, with updates on my art, workshops, speaking engagements and spiritual counseling.

   …and remember, we're ALL healers!

Contents

DEDICATION		iii
A NOTE ABOUT THIS BOOK		iv
TABLE OF CONTENTS		v
FOREWORD		vi
INTRODUCTION		1
PROLOGUE		4
CHAPTER		
1	Lizards	8
2	Heroes	17
3	Moments	27
4	Crash Course	45
5	Tovarruvias	58
6	Getting Across	64
7	The Other Side of the Tracks	74
8	Gathering Forces	82
9	Standing Orders	100
10	Suspended	113
11	Men and Machines	131
12	Tug of War	144
13	Teaching Teresa	162
14	Last Words	173
Epilogue		182

Foreword to the 1st Edition

This book is a Collector's Edition. It is the only edition where I will have written my own Foreword. The next edition will be introduced by someone who I am yet to meet, but has been moved so by the work he/she will feel compelled to contribute. It will be a surprise to us all!

Mail me your copy and include a return envelope with postage. I'll be happy to sign it on this page in thanks for helping me to get this work off the ground.

Blessings to you and yours!

INTRODUCTION:
Anyone get the number of that truck?

In the mid nineteen-eighties I left my twelve year career in Emergency Medical Services. It was as if I had broken free from the bottom of a huge vehicle that snagged and dragged me fifty twisty-turny miles across the city and into the sticks after I accidentally tripped and fell under it.

There I was, sitting on the roadside, intact and not knowing why! Strewn behind me were chunks that had been shorn away from the core of my humanity. Paradoxically, the protection they provided saved me, yet, in order for me to go on living; I could not pick them up again.

I rode the first wave of Mobile Intensive Care Unit Paramedics in the United States. I was thrust into a newly formed profession. It was a reflection of an approximate two decade shift in allopathic medicine from accessible, personal connection-driven, hands-on patient "care" to a costly, litigation-driven, technologically oriented, impersonal delivery system. The human body became a vehicle to repair, and mechanics were created to use the tools that were invented to do the repairs. We who embodied this transition had no idea how we reflected these changes.

Emergency medical care and transportation of the sick and injured switched from "load and go" to "stand and deliver." The idea was that now, we could really save lives because, after all, we had the tools! Many of us in the field had spent years barely having an effect in serious medical or traumatic situations. Once given the chance, we stretched every rule in the book to get more tools and use them more often.

The systems of which I was a part seemed to be grudgingly adapting to a sudden wave of technology that placed a bunch of renegade kids into positions of high responsibility. It seemed important that those who actually delivered the care and sometimes saved lives be kept under control because if they had their way, it would cost a lot more money!

That was all about politics. Much of my time was spent lobbying for recognition of the profession and its practitioners. It was all about enabling medics to do the best job they could. That battle rages on, I was just one of its very first casualties! That happened right after my greatest victory, the formation of the first AFL-CIO affiliation with an association of EMS professionals; the California Paramedics Association.

But all that was just the setting. A deeper and more personal drama unfolded within it; the conflicts between my head and heart.

After I got burned by and then burned out on the politics and left the field I was compelled to fulfill a sacred obligation; to articulate my experience of this extraordinary world that rocked *all* aspects of my life. As a writer, to really capture it was too rich a challenge to pass up!

At first, the story came visually. I wrote a screenplay. It consumed my life for nine years. The result was a film; *Healer*. It opened the *1994 Santa Barbara International Film Festival*. David McCallum and Tobey Maguire were in it. It was stillborn, but that's another story.

In describing my personal journey, the movie was Level I; there was territory yet to cover. Still enthralled by what I discovered about my humanity, I wanted to bring readers into an expanded experience.

My *life* had been enriched by my vulnerabilities, tears, pain, and doubts; things rarely spoken about by EMS and allied professionals. *But I had gone through a major learning curve to get there!* I experienced enhanced states of consciousness and emotion while doing the work, yet I *still* delivered the goods! How could I show that as well?

I watched so many of my peers burn out, in large part because they choked on their silence; they got shook and believed they had no where to bring their trauma. Somehow, I wanted to open a door so in the future it would be okay for them to share what shook them with each other. Who else could understand better?

When I first started to face my personal demons I began taking notes. I turned them into true short stories recapturing the emotional territory I traveled through. At the time, I was working things out. The end result was I did gain a greater appreciation for and understanding of my place in the battleground between life and death.

A thread running through the stories was that something cold was warming up. I wondered about that. Did I have a linear progression from human to Flesh Mechanic? I dropped the short story format to build a narrative in book form, covering my whole career. I failed. My progress was through an accumulation of random moments. I committed to honestly capture the experience, but I had to find another way.

In the meantime, media treatment of the profession barely acknowledged the incredible *depth* of the human experiences in it; how the work magnifies personal struggles. Literature echoed Jack Webb's *EMERGENCY!* TV show of the 1970's, reflecting Johnny and Roy, cop/firemen clones with technical expertise but nary an ounce of wonder in their bones. Reality TV and movies

Moments in the Death of a Flesh Mechanic...a healer's rebirth

were much the same; broadly portraying medics in the Flesh Mechanic stage and on the way to burnout, if not already there.

I found no fault with the honesty, yet I knew I could expand the conversation. My story was different but I wasn't sure how to tell it so people in the medical profession could hear.

Who I am today lives vibrantly because the Flesh Mechanic I was had died through harrowing moments that chipped into my protective shell, liberating the very human healer inside! This was a tale even I hadn't seen until going back once again to the short stories. Santa Barbara County at the mid-point of my career was the setting.

That young medic thought he was telling us about a professional thrust into moments that shook his understanding of the world and his place in it. But what I heard in his voice was a Flesh Mechanic telling us about the world that formed him, times when the healer in him was assaulted and he put on armor to protect it, and then moments that ripped through that armor exposing a human being who happened to be a medic.

This final work is a collaborative effort. The author is a man who helped someone half his age to tell the story of how the author was born. He worked with the young man's material so both could better understand what happened. Here is their mutual exploration of the wonders of heart, head, death, life, flesh, spirit, judgment and action. It is told through true stories of a man navigating amidst their struggles.

Moments in the Death of a Flesh Mechanic...a healer's rebirth has a very modest agenda; it was written to encourage medics of all kinds to expand their conversations to include things that rock them *as if such things really mattered!*

I encourage *all* who read this to make sacred and safe space for yourself and your peers to explore the more disturbing aspects of your *lives*. Note, I said *lives*, not work. We are human beings experiencing our lives within the context of the jobs we do. That is my point. Being a paramedic happened to be the metaphor I was given to illustrate it.

If this work is any testament, the time will come when your persistence in exploring yourself as a human being will create something useful for others. Why else go through it?

Russ Reina, Maui, HI

Feel free to drop me a line at moments@firetender.org

Prologue

It was 1973 and I had just been released from Riker's Island prison.

A year before, I was a student at a nursing school in Queens, NY, one of two males amidst a sea of 365 women. I was arrested and convicted for "*attempted criminal sale of a dangerous drug*" a 4th degree felony. I *tried* to sell three ounces of marijuana to an undercover cop. He was a friend of a friend; long-haired and happy to toke.

I spent four months in a residential, behavior-modification style cult of a drug rehabilitation program run by ex-heroin addicts. It helped me avoid serving 8 to 15 years. The NYC court system was being run tight as a drum, having just suffered the Serpico scandals where the Police were found to be wholly corrupt, but that's another story!

On sentencing, I was pulled from the program and served four months, five days and 12 hours in New York City prisons. Back to the program after release, I stayed for four more months. One night, I "split" by squeezing out a bathroom window. I was battered but not broken.

There's a curse that's placed on you in the prison system. From the day you enter until the day you leave, you hear, "You'll be back!" In New York City the recidivism rate was 87 percent. Even though I was in for just *trying* to sell marijuana, the odds were against me. I was told this time and again and I bought in to it. It took me the next three and a half years before I was able to leave my palpable paranoia behind me.

After being discharged I got an old job back in the operating room of a Hospital in Flushing, Queens. At night I'd sit at home, afraid to go out for fear of "falling." Not back into drugs, but into jail. I knew I was being watched and was primed for something to go wrong. I had time on my hands with nothing to do. I decided I needed an outlet. A couple of blocks from my fourth-story walk-up pillbox of an apartment stood the Flushing Community Volunteer Ambulance Corps (FCVAC). They had a sign in the window: "Volunteers needed."

I was not particularly drawn to ambulance work; the important thing was structure. I filled out an application, and there it was, the magic question:

Moments in the Death of a Flesh Mechanic...a healer's rebirth

"Have you ever been convicted of a crime?" I decided not to lie. Soon, I got my response; I was rejected. That brought me to the most important decision I've ever made in my life.

If I did not stand up to the FCVAC, I'd be (in jailhouse terms) "bending over" for everyone challenging me for the rest of my life. I could not back down. While I began taking Red Cross (American National Red Cross – ANRC today) courses, I wrote letters, submitted references and had meetings and interviews with each member and committee they had for a while. Finally, they let me in.

The members of the FCVAC met me as a person and took a gamble. To their credit, and with all my thanks and respect, the FCVAC welcomed me into a career that has defined every day of my life since!

In their converted Cadillac hearses I learned the trade. The staccato bursts of ambulance calls, each with a beginning, middle and end playing out in about forty minutes, appealed to my Gemini nature.

Soon, it became my obsession to become a paramedic. The profession was brand new, it had an air of drama and danger, and you could actually save lives, which wasn't what was happening in the back of those hearses! *There was something very seductive and exciting about working in death's neighborhood and having the weapons to fight it!*

New York State had a program reserved for a select cadre of fire department personnel. I found pilot programs in Maryland, Florida, Washington State and California. Maryland was strictly for volunteers, Washington and California too foreign, but Florida, with programs going in the private sector, seemed like my best bet. My parents and best friends from high school were living in the Orlando area also.

Without job prospects, I moved and found a county with a new paramedic program. As an Emergency Medical Technician (EMT) with operating room and ambulance experience, I got a job as Emergency Medical Technologist in an emergency room in New Smyrna Beach, a half hour south of Daytona in Volusia County.

I weaseled my way into the local private ambulance service where I got my first paid medic job: *24 hours a day, five days a week at $600 a month!* My partners and I were given a house, an ambulance, and an area to cover of about 15,000 people; most of them were retired. One-third of our work was hauling dead bodies for local funeral homes!

We were in a "satellite office" of Beacon Ambulance, whose base station, in Daytona Beach, had five ambulances available for duty. There were four other one-ambulance satellites in the 200-square-mile county. I averaged about twenty emergency calls a week; a medium workload. As a rookie, some days I worked with Henry, an EMT, on others with Riley, who just completed the county's first paramedic course. Each was experienced. I was still a wide-eyed kid in the learning curve at the "conscious incompetence" stage. I leaned on them.

I found myself thrust into moments where, in the absence of therapies to offer, all I'd have left was connection. I saw how much power a medic has to actually influence the course of recovery of a human being. There were times I was in awe and tears at the miracles of which I had been a part. Following my feelings in *how* I handled a call became the most important tool I carried in my limited bag of tricks.

I got into the third class for paramedics (the company didn't send anyone to the second). It lasted a year. Each weekday morning I'd start the day in Daytona (Halifax Hospital Medical Center) getting classroom and clinical training. By 1:00 p.m., I'd be back on duty.

The system had a unique component to it. If I learned about a technique or procedure in my Clinicals at 10:00 a.m. and practiced it, as long as I was partnered with a paramedic that evening, I could use it on a patient *that very day*. I was in heaven! At the same time, I was still struggling to get my functional EMT skills up to par.

The day I graduated, however, something clicked: "Oh My GOD!" I thought, "These people's lives are in *my* hands now!" It wasn't until that moment I realized I had no more room to be casual. This was very serious. Until then, it was still a vehicle helping me have an exciting life while keeping me out of trouble in a somnolent community.

Once a paramedic, I had to push my edges and develop skills you'd expect to learn in a field with far more intrigue, like being a mercenary! I would have used any tool at my disposal to make sure the program continued. When I say everything I learned, I learned in the back of an ambulance, I'm not kidding!

The program was a completely new way of thinking and acting. It had to be *sold*. Overcoming the skepticism of a populace who only knew and understood ambulance personnel as "drivers" whose job it was to "load and go" was an indispensable part of the job.

The scrutiny was relentless. You were only as good as your last call. A string of well-run calls meant nothing if you came in with an unsuccessful I.V. Understanding the system meant nothing to the Sheriff if, in that moment, he simply wanted the collapsed man in the bar OUT!

Just when I thought I was accepted as a valuable member of the health care team, I found myself defending everything I did. In the beginning, everyone dealing with the new industry kept the pressure up. Accusations flew about companies using paramedic services for the profits. Often, I didn't know if I'd have a job the next morning due to company squabbles with the county, budget cutbacks, or even bad press!

There was no guidebook showing the kinds of things I had to face in this arena. Proportionally, the number of people who I saved was small, yet, I had

Moments in the Death of a Flesh Mechanic…a healer's rebirth

to promote paramedic services like a carnival barker, all the while knowing most of what I did was haul bodies from the hospital to the nursing home and too often, to the morgue or funeral home. Occasionally, I'd get crack at grabbing someone from the jaws of death.

And then, there were moments that came when they pleased and from out of nowhere; like ghouls from the darkness in a haunted house ride. I was never prepared. *I knew I'd be exposed to others' pain, scenes of destruction, my own limitations and emotional, philosophical, psychic and spiritual conflicts, but I had no idea there were so many varieties!*

Developing into a professional was an arduous journey through my own personal hell. Character defects, personal limits in my beliefs or ability to act would emerge; sometimes with devastating consequences.

The more technical information I had to absorb, the less room I had for my human experience. I was knocked off balance when I'd pause and consider. There's no time for that at first. So I did the most common thing; I distanced myself from my internal life.

Working effectively meant not being surprised. I took every opportunity to insulate myself from feeling the relentless assaults I was subject to. There were more of them once I became a paramedic. My emotions became the only unpredictable pieces of equipment I carried!

By the time I arrived in Santa Barbara County, CA, where most of the action of this book takes place, I had at least five years experience in ambulance work under my belt. I was relatively comfortable, if not cocky handling my responsibilities. My skin was thick, too.

Still, it all was an experiment in danger of failing; not only the profession, but my involvement in it as well. Like I had seen with so many others of my peers, there was likely to be a call out there with my name on it, and it could be the one to cause me to bolt!

The young ex-con had grown into a professional! As I had done so, almost imperceptibly, I also had donned thick layers of protection.

Paradoxically, the more proficient and experienced I became in the work, the more I began to rely once again on my feelings. When that crack widened, new challenges stepped in. For the first time in my career my defenses started getting in my way.

That was about the time the Flesh Mechanic I had become began to clash with a new human being who was intent on emerging.

Chapter One

LIZARDS

Why, I don't know, but in the past year, the subject hadn't come up. Maybe the medics in the North County were green. Or maybe it was because there just weren't enough of those calls to make it an issue. Regardless, there sat my new partner, behind the wheel of the ambulance on my first working day in south Santa Barbara County, and he was bitching about having to haul lizards.

"What'd you say?" I asked.

"Lizards," Jake replied, "I hate coming in and first thing in the morning I've got to haul a lizard to the nursing home."

"That's incredible!" I was truly amazed. "Never worked in the south did ya? You know, like the Civil War-type south?"

"Surely not," he answered, "Santa Barbara every minute since I started ambulance six years ago."

"Un-fuckin' believable," I exclaimed, "I've been in California a year now and this is the first...Shit...I thought we only called 'em Lizards in Florida!"

"Well," Jake said, "I don't know. Here, we always called them that. And nobody's brought that word up here from down there because you're the only one from down there who's come up here."

This was weird. An unusual piece of EMT slang from the Deep South was the same terminology used on the other end of the continent!

"Why do you," I asked, sensing fun, "call them Lizards, here?"

"Well, hell," Jake turned and looked at me like I was loco, "look at 'em." He put his face into a vacant stare. "They got that flap of skin," he drew an imaginary line in the air from the tip of his chin down to the top of his breastbone about two inches from his own skin, "it hangs like this here. Then they got those gnarly corrugated circles under their eyes. When you touch them, it feels like scrambled eggs sitting on the stove for a day — like a lizard, of course."

Moments in the Death of a Flesh Mechanic...a healer's rebirth

Halfway in, tears filled my eyes I was laughing so hard.

"We called 'em that in Florida," I said, "for a different reason."

"Go ahead," Jake started the ambulance. We weren't in a rush.

"You know," I started, "when you first push the gurney through the doors into the main hall of the nursing home? What happens?"

Jake thought a moment and replied, "They look. They stare."

"And what does it look like?" I asked. I started to paint the picture with my hands; I'm Italian, I do that. "All these little gray heads pop up out of nooks and crannies. A head comes up behind a chair. Another one peeks out from behind a lamp or a bookcase. Soon as they get a whiff that someone new is coming in, or someone sick or dead is goin' out, or someone's gonna be kidnapped and sent to somewhere worse, those little heads pop out. But they don't want to be *it* so they wait and watch."

"You're right," said Jake. His eyes lit up enthusiastically. "They hide and peek and check you out until they're sure it ain't *them* you're coming for..."

"When they know they're safe," I finished, "WHOOSH, the little gray heads are gone. They pop back into their holes; like lizards in a rock pile!"

We both started to laugh, but then, simultaneously stopped. Perhaps we were sick of it. Jake put the unit into gear and we jumped out of the driveway. The jolt back to sobriety reminded me of a call I had in Florida.

I was an EMT riding in the back with an old woman who was on her way to a nursing home. She rambled on about peach trees and gardens and hedges, making wide sweeps with her arms as if in the midst of the scene she was describing. She was absolutely there! Judging by the tone of her voice and her words, she was back in her childhood. I was completely fascinated. At one point, she threw her head back with glee and exclaimed to me, holding out her hand for me to see, "Aren't these *the* most gorgeous lemons you've ever seen?"

She was so thrilled I burst out laughing, genuinely appreciating the moment, and her. In a burst of movement, she drew her arm back, straightened herself out on the gurney and, looking me right in the eyes as serious as cancer, slowly said, "It's easy for you to laugh. It's hard for me. I just wait and wait."

"I hate starting my day off in one of those places," Jake said.

"Yeah," was my reply.

I came to Florida from New York after doing volunteer work in the Flushing Community Volunteer Ambulance Corps (FCVAC). I ended up switching from a compact, city system covering a population of about 100,000 people to a rural area with 15,000 people. Worse than that, 80% of the residents were retired. The remaining 20 percent were employed in some aspect of serving them.

Many of the aging and aged were still spry, but there was a sizable number who were far less fortunate. There were all sorts of "homes" available for them; board and care, rest, convalescent, and nursing, making it rather clear that no one related to them was actually keeping them "home". By far, the worst of these were the nursing homes.

A lot of their residents had simply been discarded; remanded to an institution. It didn't seem most residents were *living* there. "Existed" would be more of an accurate word. For these places were the last stop before oblivion for those whose bodies would not give up, even long after their spirits and minds seemed to have evacuated their shells.

The sad thing was none were really sick enough to die soon and no one was healthy or robust enough to take care of themselves or have anything like an active life. The nursing homes on my beat housed bodies that lingered: Period.

At first, forty per cent of my work time was spent transporting old folk; from the nursing homes to clinics and hospitals and back, or to mortuaries. At times from their own or children's homes and right in to nursing homes — sometimes kicking and screaming! Many with minds left understood the nursing home would be their last stop on this earth.

The majority of the nursing homes were geared toward custody and maintenance rather than rehabilitation or improvement. Where I worked, nursing homes kept the body breathing, fed, clean, and peaceable through pharmacology. No one was discharged from a nursing home with more than a few breaths left to breathe.

I didn't need to ask Jake if I could expect much of the same here. I'd know soon. Our headquarters was strategically placed to allow us to get to the sites of these non-emergency, "Code One" transfers within a couple of minutes.

In Santa Barbara at that time, an average weekday would yield four pre-scheduled Code One, non-emergency transfers per unit. As long as good relationships with hospitals, clinics and nursing homes were cultivated and maintained, the company could count on that income. Transfers were crucial to the survival of most private ambulance companies. That's true today, as well.

Ironically, a string of emergencies could delay the transport of a routine pre-scheduled transfer and hurt the company. If things like that happened often enough, it would mean the facility would stop using the service. This loss of steady income could be devastating. Much care was taken to assure Code Ones were attended to properly and promptly. Woe be to the discourteous, lackadaisical, or late medic! The company's life was dependent on Code One.

We pulled the ambulance into the parking lot of the home; just a few blocks from Cottage Hospital, the main receiving facility for the area. The rectangular brick building was consistent with the other fortress-like structures that I was used to. I reflexively prepared for battle.

Moments in the Death of a Flesh Mechanic...a healer's rebirth

"Medic Three's 10-97," Jake spoke into the mic, letting dispatch know we had arrived, "what'd you say that patient's name was and where's he going?"

"Alden Baxter: transfer to Cottage Hospital, 4N," she replied.

"Ten-four," Jake replied and hung up the mic. "You know," he offered, "It used to be I'd pray for a Code Three to come down. I'd drop the Lizard, go in-service and handle it. I don't do that now; caught too much flack. I let dispatch figure it out. I see the business sense of the whole thing, you know?"

"Yeah, you're right," I had to agree, although reluctantly.

I, too, had once thought that to be a paramedic was devoting one's all to saving lives. It wasn't so. To be a paramedic meant being a vehicle for income for the company so the company could provide you the tools and opportunity to act like a paramedic once in a while. Serving as a part-time taxi driver for recumbent individuals was the only way to reach all the people in an area. It had taken me years to get the concept straight in my head that, indeed, my ability to contribute altruistically was built on my support of the profit motive.

We took the gurney and went in through one of the back doors of the nursing home. It was 7:30 in the morning, so there was only one old lady tapping her way down the hallway in her wheelchair. She must have been a "Screamer." That's someone who wakes up and screams to high heaven until he or she has been taken out of bed.

This was all too familiar territory. I started my medical career in 1969 as a nurse's aide. I did the work, and the nurse pushed pills, of which Thorazine, that efficient pacifier, was the most bountiful! I knew in an hour the halls would turn into a gauntlet of wheelchair bound, blank-faced old folk. Those who could get around on their own would not be out until about 10:00 a.m. — it would take them that long to get themselves together enough to greet the day.

Nursing home routine was simple and grueling: 7:15 a.m., breakfast trays out; 8:20, finish spoon-feeding your fourth patient; 8:25, pick up trays; 8:30, fill cart with washcloths, towels, diapers, and soap; 8:35, start working on your patients. Then, crank 'em out — get the bodies out of bed. The ratio was one nurse's aide to 10 patients — that's cardiac crippled, stroked out, diabetic or traumatic amputees, or generally debilitated bed and wheelchair-bound patients. It was tough, assembly-line work until about 11:30 and still, one or two would have to stay in bed until after lunch.

One-third were showered, the rest given quick bed baths, diapered, transferred into wheelchairs and pushed into the hall or down the corridor into the "Rec. Room" and placed in front of a TV. Moving around flesh; I hated it.

For the longest time, when asked what my job was, I'd reply, "Why, I'm a professional ass wiper!" I was glad to be out of it, though I questioned if I'd ever be free.

This Santa Barbara "home" was not much different from others I had known, although these hallways felt like confusingly articulated, antiseptic-smelling catacombs. At the nurse's station, I was not surprised to see a young, very good-looking nurse fiddling with a huge, wide tray filled with paper cups holding pills, pills, and more pills. Nursing homes were good money for a fresh graduate.

The sad part was, etched into her face was the same furrowed brow and mechanically focused eyes prevalent on burned-out nurses more than twice her age. Without looking up from her organizational nightmare, she simply pointed to her left and said, "Four-eighteen."

Jake asked for the patient's chart so he could copy some information on to our "trip-sheet" while I took the gurney over to the room. When I entered, the lights were still off. Not wanting to make a big deal of waking up everyone in the room, I just rolled the gurney in. As my eyes started to adjust, I could see that only one of the beds in the room had a body in it. Without bothering to go back to the light switch, I brought the gurney alongside the bed.

My ears recognized something; a rhythm. It sent off an alarm in my head. Focusing on what I was hearing, I backed up to the light switch and turned it on. I stood and stared at what I could see now was a man in the bed. I tried to link what I saw with what I heard to confirm or deny my suspicions.

At first I was blinded; only the man's breathing sounds came through clearly. I heard two quick and sharp intakes of breath. And then there was silence. My eyes were now seeing the man's chest. It was clear there was no movement. So, I did what I sensed I was supposed to do. I waited. Wasn't I supposed to spring into action? After all, it was the airway. Not really. By that point in my career, I was learning to respond to what I felt over what I had been taught.

After a few seconds, the chest moved slightly, and the man sucked in a small breath: A shallow exhalation; a pause; another movement and another breath — this one slightly deeper. An exhalation, a shorter pause, movement, a stronger intake of air; the words "stair-step respirations" popped in to my mind.

Then, my eyes realized the man's lips were blue, his face in pallor, and he was unconscious. I had noticed, but I had to get rid of my preconception that this was a routine transfer before I could really *see* what was there.

This was supposed to be a transfer, I thought. Hell, this guy's circling the drain! "Christalmighty," I whispered quietly to myself and then yelled out as loudly as I could, "Jake...*Jake*, get-in-here- Now!"

Footsteps came running. Another set, less resonant, lagged behind. I started to slap together an assessment. Naturally, responding to a non-emergency transfer, my bag of tricks was still sitting in the rig!

I jerkily reached across and my hand inadvertently rubbed up against a bloody big lump on the back of his head by the base of his skull. I felt for his carotid artery and felt a weak pulse, almost indiscernible. Jake entered. By now, my eyes were hopping from place to place, trying to put the pieces together.

"Jake," I called out, "this guy's Cheynne-Stoking!" Cheynne-Stokes respiration is a sign of serious head injury or stroke; the last phase of breathing before it's all over. Breaths are shallow and far between at first. They increase in depth and frequency until suddenly the patient goes apneic — stops breathing. When and if the cycle resumes is a crapshoot. The nurse sauntered in.

"I thought this was a Code-One transfer?" Jake asked the nurse evenly — diplomatically, yet, with a touch of accusation. "You called in for a routine transfer. You said it wasn't urgent."

"The *other* RN," the nurse explained, "said an aide told her he wasn't so good. She looked in, called his doctor, and he said that he'd admit him. I..."

"You better just get the crash cart in here," Jake interrupted forcefully. As soon as she left the room, I told Jake what I had found.

"This guy took a dive some time last night," I said. "Look, there's some blood on the floor; and on the bed there. It smeared where they put him back in. He's got a big lump down by the base of the skull. I feel crepitus; crackly, probably a depressed skull fracture. Neck seems okay, but no telling."

"Let's intubate, breathe him, start an IV and get him out to the rig." Jake offered. A nurse and an orderly came in pulling a large, red, Craftsman™ tool cabinet behind them. The nurse fumbled with the keys.

"Was there a note on his chart not to do heroics?" I asked aloud while Jake took a laryngoscope blade and handle from a drawer.

"No," replied the nurse as she let some fluid run through the IV line that she had just attached to an old-style glass bottle, "he was just admitted a few days ago. The family hadn't decided."

"That's great!" cursed Jake. Not at her statement, but at the light at the tip of the curved metal laryngoscope blade. It did not go on when the blade was snapped into position on the handle. Apparently, its batteries were dead.

Jake threw the laryngoscope down to the foot of the bed while I inserted a needle into a vein in the man's forearm. Jake took out a thinner endotracheal tube than the first. He spread some K-Y® jelly on its tip, poised it point down just above the man's nostril and waited.

Jake counted. He waited until the man was at his strongest intake of air. Then, while positioning the man's head and manipulating the slender tube, he pushed it into the man's nostril, down into his throat, past his open epiglottis, between his vocal cords and into the windpipe. It's called a *blind*, nasotrachael intubation.

I quickly finished anchoring the IV line to the man's arm and, grabbing my stethoscope (always around my neck), listened to the man's chest as Jake began administering oxygen by an outdated, military style Ambu-bag and oxygen cylinder bungeed on to the crash cart.

If you intubate too deeply, the tube will go down the right fork of the trachea and only the right lung will inflate. You must get it just right. Jake got it just right; I was impressed. As soon as I gave him the nod, Jake injected five cc's of air into the tube's wrap-around inflatable cuff. The air expanded a membrane around the rigid tube, anchoring it in the man's windpipe. As soon as I was sure it was stable, I moved to the cardiac monitor, also strapped to the cart with bungee cords.

Thank God, I was familiar with this dinosaur of a monitor. It was one of the first — a Lifepak 2™. Weighing in at around 40 pounds, it was three times the bulk and weight of our Life-Pak 5™.

The nurse called out a BP of 80 over 70. One more bad sign in a series of bad signs getting worse. The closer the upper number is to the lower number in traumatic emergencies, the more likely it is that blood pressure will quickly go crashing through the floor; in seconds perhaps!

We weren't very encouraged by what we saw on the monitor, either. It showed sinus bradycardia; a very slow rhythm. There were frequent wide and irregular beats popping off between those slow beats — premature ventricular contractions (PVCs), a sure sign of decreased oxygen assimilation. The problem was, we could eliminate the PVCs by administering Lidocaine, but if we eliminated them, there wouldn't be enough beats left to keep blood flowing!

Still, for a disaster, this call was running like clockwork. Both Jake and I knew that any other therapy would have to happen in the rig...and fast!

We loosened the sheet from under the patient. The one thing done right was the patient's sheets were perfectly tight! We jerked him to the gurney. Everything happened so reflexively. Not until we lowered the gurney to half-height to make it easier to work on the man did I look around me for a second and exclaim to myself, "What's the use?"

But then, images flashed: A restless man; an unsecured guardrail; a twist; a turn; his upper torso flips off the bed; he grabs at the air, too late; the back of his head hits the floor with a loud CRAACKK; the rest of him follows. Time passes. An aide appears panics and leaves. Two aides struggle and lift him into bed. One raises the guardrail, the other tucks in the sheets. They leave.

I felt a sinking feeling in my stomach. I didn't have time to ponder why; the line on the monitor went flat. Not erratically jerky, which is reversible by defibrillation (shocking the heart with 400 joules of electricity), but flat; asystole — no electrical activity at all. And then, the man stopped breathing.

From reflex, I began chest compressions. If this was a heart problem, we could have used a battery of drugs on him. It was not. This was a traumatic head injury. He may as well have been decapitated.

Moments in the Death of a Flesh Mechanic...a healer's rebirth

Jake pulled the electrode wires out of the bulky monitor, interposed a couple of breaths through the ET tube with the Ambu-bag, and started to push the gurney out of the room. We were out of there.

I maintained a rhythm of compressions as best I could while stepping sideways with the gurney. We made a right turn, and the nurse came running out after us yelling, "NO; the other way!"

We changed direction and headed down another hallway, and I could hear Screamers. There were many wheelchair-bound patients in the hallway. Some others craned their necks out from the safety of their rooms to see.

He was heavier than I thought. While lifting the gurney into the ambulance, Jake jerked up faster than I, and the man tilted heavily toward me. My back wrenched. As soon as I got into the unit, Jake slammed the door shut, got in the cab and took off. I began one-man CPR. Jake told Dispatch to notify Cottage Hospital ER to "prepare for a Code Blue; quick! We're one minute out."

We were met at the emergency room bay by a contingent of nurses and orderlies. They swiftly helped us unload and get the man into the cardiac room. A doctor was ready for us. While I continued compressions and a respiratory therapist took over breathing, the doctor palpated the back of his skull, shined a light into his eyes to check pupil reactivity and glanced at the monitor screen that had been hooked up to our electrodes. He motioned me to stop.

"His doctor called in," the ER doc said. "He said, 'If it looks bad, let him go'. Let him go." So we did.

There was a sudden sense of silence and emptiness where once had been rhythmical movement, internal counting ("one-one-thousand, two-one-thousand, three-one-thousand..." with each compression according to the American Heart Association standards at the time), and what I realized had been my own labored breathing. My hands had stopped compressing the man's chest, but I let them linger for a moment, palms down. I spread my fingers and just held them there. There was nothing I could connect with but clammy flesh. I picked my hands up and away from his chest and walked away.

While Jake filled out the call sheet, which lists times, scene details, physical evaluations, vital signs, therapies and other data, I filled out an incident report. This was going to be a coroner's case!

"You know," I said to Jake, "I didn't realize how great it was not to have many Fig Farms in the area. While I was in the North County last year, there was only one; hardly ran a call in it. In Florida, Christ, we'd have one a month that'd go sour like this. Just like this."

"All I know is," Jake said seriously, "all I do these days is haul Lizards. It's beginning to look to me like that's all you can look forward to when you get that old...some snot-nosed kid wiping your butt in the nursing home and then abusing you. It's pretty desperate; being nothing; meaning nothing."

"Yeah," I commented, "we live long enough, that's where we're gonna end up, huh?"

"That's pretty scary, isn't it?" Jake continued. "Hell. We did good by this guy. Maybe I'm starting to get older. Used to be I looked at it this way," Jake took in a deep breath and eyed me as if he were debating whether it was safe to reveal himself; "...you did your best on Lizards for one reason..."

"Practice," I interrupted. "I know the drill." Get your skills up on the unsalvageable so when you get a real call, you've got it all down.

I suddenly felt embarrassed.

"You ever admit that to someone on the outside?" he asked.

"Yeah...right!" I replied.

"Me neither," Jake said, smiling.

"This guy wasn't practice," I said. And then I asked, "You?"

"Nope." Jake answered me so quickly I was startled. He continued: "Maybe we were the only people in the world who gave a shit if the old fart lived or died."

"Maybe," I agreed. "It looked like someone needed to."

"Sometimes," Jake looked me right in the eyes, "I hope I've still got the strength and the balls to pull the trigger as soon as I know I'm heading for a place like that."

"Anyone would who sees what we see," I said.

As I finished, the handheld radio on my belt went off with a tone. "Medic Three," said the dispatcher, "prepare to copy a call."

We looked at each other. It was obvious Jake's wheels were turning, too. Somehow, if this was a Lizard run, we'd damn well weasel our way out of it.

Chapter Two
HEROES

"What are *you* here for?"

The old, oversized woman, dressed in an even more oversized flannel night gown covered by an alpaca wool sweater and wearing fuzzy house slippers stood at her front door and challenged us.

"We got an emergency call here," I stammered. Vapor from the cold billowed out of my mouth. "Didn't you call 9-1-1?"

"Me?" She looked at me as if I was stupid. "No. You think maybe," she raised her arms and asked the four winds, "it was my daughter that called?"

"I don't know, Lady," said my partner, Drew, rubbing his hands together impatiently; "all I know is we got a call for a 'man down'."

Neither of us was going to back down easily on this call. It was designed for us. Besides, it was pretty cold standing on that porch.

"This is 12 Graciosa Road, isn't it?" I asked.

"Yes, it is," was her reply. She took in a deep breath that helped her massive body fill up the doorway even more.

"Well, then," I firmly continued, "we *have to* come in."

I fidgeted uncomfortably in the cold. Carrying our APCOR™ cardiac telemetry radio in one hand and gripping the cold handle of our drug box in the other, I just wanted to get inside.

The woman waffled between resignation and defiance. Her face changed expression a couple of times as if she were debating with herself. This call was getting pretty weird fast. If we were wrong, we were bullying the poor woman; not good for public relations. But if there was something going on, we were wasting precious time.

"Lady," Drew tried in his most professional manner, but I could tell his patience was wearing thin, "we received a call for a man who collapsed at this address. We can't leave here without knowing firsthand everything is okay."

There was no way we were going to walk away. This call was a fluke; it was meant to save *our* asses.

We had been sitting at our quarters in the volunteer fire station of the little town of Orcutt for almost 60 hours — two and one-half days of our three-day shift. The whole weekend had gone by without a call. Not even a move-up to cover someone else's area while they ran calls.

Worse was that we were in the middle of a cold spell; cold for Southern California, anyway. It wasn't comfortable to leave the station. It wasn't comfortable to stay there, either. Its ramshackle heater was barely a step better than newspaper on fire in a garbage can!

Bored would not even describe it. About an hour and a half ago, after we had risen from a three-hour nap, we decided to go cruising.

We stepped into the unit and went 10-8 (in service) and told dispatch we were going grocery shopping and one of us would be available in the rig to take calls that we really didn't think would come.

One thing led to another, and before we knew it, we were five miles out of town, following some godforsaken trail up and over a set of hills into an oil field lease off of Highway 101. The poor dirt excuse for a road wound around a series of green scrub pine covered hillocks looking like gumdrops just plopped down on the flat landscape.

We hadn't thought twice about what we were doing until about the one-hour mark. Dispatch, busy with calls in the southern part of the county, wasn't keeping track of us. They had probably forgotten there was even a north county, given how slow things had been lately.

As if we had each heard the other's internal time clock ticking more loudly, Drew and I looked at each other, and we knew we better get our butts back. The adrenaline rush we had been missing over the last couple of days bubbled up inside us. We were lost!

It seemed reasonable to pick our way across the oil field roads until we made it to Highway 135. We had a map from the fire station. Jabbering away while I drove and Drew navigated, however, we passed a number of forks and, amidst our distraction, had not kept track.

The sun dropped below the horizon like a stone. We had to strain our eyes to see. The unit's headlights were no help because of the transition from color to gray. Drew came out with a brilliant observation.

"All those cars we saw before," he said, "just as we pulled in? Those were the roughnecks going home for the day."

He was right. We had completely disrupted our wake-sleep cycle. Mid-afternoon naps followed by ice cream and TV binges lasting until 3:00 a.m. had completely screwed up our sense of time.

Moments in the Death of a Flesh Mechanic...a healer's rebirth

We found ourselves in the middle of nowhere with no one to guide us and the lights sinking fast! With a fixed opening between the cab of the ambulance and the patient compartment, even the rig's heater was hard-pressed to keep us warm.

We paused by some cows standing in an open pasture threading its way in between a number of oil pumps. One option was to backtrack until we found a familiar landmark. Unfortunately, the only landmarks there were the oil pumps. In the dim light, one was indistinguishable from the next. We decided instead to push on toward the following set of hills and take a left at the fork.

After that set, we took a jagged left and went over to another set of hills and decided to try them. On the other side, finding still another set before us, we decided to skip them and head to the right. Then we came across a group of black-and-white cows who were huddling close together, snorting steam and chewing their cuds.

"They look familiar, don't they?" Drew said. "Cows don't go very fast or very far, do they?"

"How should I know?" I snapped; "I grew up in Brooklyn!"

Sure enough, we were back at the first set of hills. Maybe it was the second set; I didn't know. This time, instead of making a left, I made a right to the top of a very steep road that dead-ended at a series of pumps. While turning around, we spotted the highway we had been looking for. Re-oriented, I made a bee-line down the hill and drove like hell through the tight little valley.

It opened up into an open field that stretched out to a small service road that ran parallel to the highway. About a half mile ahead, we could see the lights of a couple of farm houses.

"Medic Seven," went our radio, "what's your location?"

"Oh shit..." Drew started to ask, "Where did we say..."

"Control One," I tried to deflect her. "You have something?"

"We have a call for a man down," the dispatcher replied, "at twelve Graciosa Road; a farm house. Thomas Brothers 14, D-2. ETA?"

She bought it! I looked and realized that Graciosa was the very road we were headed for. The lights ahead were the only houses on it!

"Medic Seven," I said, struggling to keep the amazement out of my voice, "is...um...we're 10-97."

"You're on the scene?" came back the dispatcher incredulously.

I handed the microphone to Drew, in part because I wanted to concentrate on sprinting the last quarter mile to the house, in part because, hell, he's my partner, and he's got to sweat a little, too!

"Affirmative," Drew said into the mic, "Um...thank you very much," and then he put the microphone back in its cradle.

"Thank you very much!" I laughed. "Good one!"

Within 15 seconds of getting the call, I pulled the ambulance into the driveway by the mailbox marked 12. That's why neither of us had any intention of leaving without a patient. Instantaneously showing up on the scene of an emergency usually elicits a "Well done; that'll look good in our response time reports!" If we left that house empty-handed, however, we wouldn't have the distraction of success to fall back on and the questions about where we had been would start coming.

The woman blocking the doorway was now looking a little sad.

"I thought my daughter," she said, "was just going to call ..."

Both my and Drew's ears perked up, but for a split second we weren't quite sure what to do. The woman went on.

"He just dropped dead." She said this so matter-of-factly it startled me. But my partner's immediate response threw me even more.

"Jesus God, lady," he said, "People just don't drop dead anymore!" And then he gently moved her to the side with his hand and walked into the house. After a slight hesitation, I followed.

It was almost as cold inside as it was outside. She followed us in and began haranguing us in what sounded like a Russian accent.

"My God," she moaned, "I told you he just dropped dead! He was 75 years old. He had the kencer. No surprise; don't you listen?"

Face down on the floor in between a low, bare coffee table and a couch, was a large man dressed in pants, shirt and a wool sports coat. Drew went to him and moved the table aside.

I put down my equipment and helped Drew carefully log-roll the man on to his back. His face was cold and blue.

The woman sat down on the couch and started nudging the man's body with her foot as she talked.

"He's dead, I tell you. Before I called my daughter, I called the doctor. I said, 'Doctor Edelman, what we've been waiting for has just happened. Gordon has passed away.'"

I tilted his head back and checked for breathing while Drew checked for a pulse.

"The doctor said," she continued, "'I'm so sorry, Velma.' That's what he said, 'I'm so sorry.'"

Drew and I looked at each other, and we knew we had each come up zero. The man sure looked dead; stiff; everything felt dead.

Moments in the Death of a Flesh Mechanic...a healer's rebirth

We were in a precarious spot. You do not automatically start resuscitative efforts: First comes the decision. If it is expected, for example, and the tacit agreement between the family and doctor is no "heroic" efforts are to be made — particularly in the case of aged patients — you run the risk of starting a commotion when you burst in and start resuscitative efforts. It's an assaultive sight, and turns what could be a peaceful transition into a traumatic experience for the family.

From what the woman said, this sounded like it might have been expected. "Might" was the operative word.

If you spend too much time screwing around and being gentle, however, the patient could cross the line and, without oxygen, get brain-dead. Then, you end up working up a corpse.

You don't want to deprive anyone of a chance. If you're going to err, it's best to do it in favor of the patient. Once you start, you're committed. It is very bad form to stop while the family is looking, sheepishly say, "Oops, we goofed," and then call the coroner. Once you start, technically, you can't stop until the doctor says stop. Functionally, once you're sure, you stop where no one can see you.

The guy looked as if he had been down a while. The scene's appearance and the woman's confusing words, coupled with the fact that we arrived immediately, made this a real borderline case. There were things to figure out and questions to ask, and it had to take place in seconds. As we opened up our equipment and got ready for the worst, we did a rapid evaluation.

I saw there was neither a walker nor a wheelchair. The man was fully dressed. I patted him below the waist and couldn't feel a bulky diaper. His shoes were tied sloppily, which led me to believe he tied them himself. No, this guy was getting around on his own power.

"You said he had cancer. Did the doctor say he was going to die from it?" I asked.

"Of course!" was her reply. "Everybody dies from the kencer! They operated on him. Cut out his...his prostrate; a year ago. I knew he'd drop dead from it soon."

"He collapsed how long ago?" Drew asked. He slid the cardiac monitor beside the man. I re-positioned his head to open his airway.

"Well," said the woman as she looked up to a clock on a mantelpiece, "he collapsed. I called the doctor. Then I called my daughter, and then you got here; maybe four, five minutes."

"Four minutes!" I exclaimed in surprise.

She nudged the body with her foot again and then continued.

"Yes," she said, "It's not proper to talk long on the phone. We were eating. He stood up. He collapsed..."

That was it; he was eating! I didn't wait for her to finish. I grabbed the man's nose, clamped it shut, tilted his head back, and taking in a deep breath, I wrapped my mouth around his tightly. I had spent so much time working with either no or ineffective airway equipment, even that far into my experience I still reflexively did unprotected mouth-to-mouth in severe circumstances.

Blowing into his mouth was like blowing into my own palm. The back pressure was so prominent, my ears popped. Now worried, I repositioned his head and tried again with the same result. I moved his head to the side and placed my hands one on top of the other just below his sternum, I pushed upward sharply — the Heimlich maneuver. No good. I repeated. No good.

This was one bitch of a Cafe Coronary!

I twisted around and lunged for the respiratory box so quickly, I knocked one of the monitor paddles out of Drew's hand. I grabbed the laryngoscope handle, a straight blade and a pair of throat forceps — huge, curved plastic tweezers. As I crawled on my knees back around to the man's head, the woman stretched out her leg to gently kick her husband's shoulder.

"The sonofabitch," she said, "I told him 'Get more insurance!'"

I positioned myself above the man's head, leaning over and looking down at his feet. I laid my tools alongside him and took his head in my hands.

"We've got V-fib," Drew called out to me. He had the man's shirt ripped open and the paddles in place.

"Let me go for this first," I said. "Charge up; be ready!"

I tilted the man's head slightly forward, opened his mouth and, picking up the laryngoscope, laid the metal blade over his tongue and down toward the back of his throat. The light at the end of the blade showed the man's epiglottis — a flap of flesh protecting the entrance to the wind pipe. What looked like another piece of flesh was behind it.

Carefully laying the tip of the blade on top of the epiglottis, I flicked it down. Yes, that was a chunk of meat in there. It was wedged between his vocal cords, distending them so the opening to his wind pipe was completely blocked. Reaching in with the plastic forceps, I was barely able to grasp a small corner of the chunk. The forceps slipped off.

"Push his gut" wasn't quite what I wanted to say, but Drew figured it out. Still holding the paddles, he took one and pressed it down and up, just below the man's sternum.

"Harder!" I called out, and as soon as Drew did so, the pressure in the man's lungs forced the meat trapped in his wind pipe to bulge out toward me. I clamped on to it as hard as I could and tugged.

A two-inch-long, half-inch-wide strip of beef popped out of the man's mouth in the forceps. I pulled out the laryngoscope blade, and positioning his neck again, blew the biggest breath I could into the man's lungs; again, and again. His chest rose perfectly each time.

I had another choice. I could intubate him first, before Drew defibrillated. By inserting a slender clear plastic tube down into his wind pipe, I could protect his airway from the aspiration of vomitus. But I didn't experience any rumbling sensations — and down that close to someone, you do — and for the fact that he hadn't vomited by now I gambled there hadn't been enough food ingested to present a problem.

It was all a crapshoot, anyway; splitting seconds. I figured we were right at the six-minute mark at that point. Six minutes since he had taken his last breath, and that was while swallowing. Once again, I wondered about just how accurate are those textbooks?

"Hit him!" I cried out as I pulled away from his body.

As Drew pressed the paddle's buttons and the body jerked from the discharge of electricity, I grabbed the Ambu-bag from the respiratory kit. I gave him a couple of breaths while the cardiac monitor line showed a big jerk, up and off the screen.

Taking an endotrachael tube out of the respiratory box, I repositioned the man's head and, using the laryngoscope again, placed the hollow tube in between his vocal cords.

The monitor line dropped down into a flat line for about three seconds. One beat came and another. I carefully anchored the tube in the man's trachea. A third beat occurred next to the second. A fourth fell right on top of that one, and then, the line started to undulate wildly, showing ventricular fibrillation — his heart went back to quivering ineffectively like a sack full of Jell-O.

Drew hit the buttons that charged the defibrillator again as I gave the man a couple more breaths. Then, quickly wrapping some tape around the tube where it came out of the man's mouth, I pressed the tape to his face, securing and stabilizing the tube.

The man's beloved got up off the couch and went to the front door. Two of the Orcutt firemen came in. One was carrying an oxygen bottle with a positive pressure valve and mask on it.

I pulled the Ambu-bag away. Drew shocked the man's heart. The fireman came up to me, took the Ambu-bag out of my hand and handed me the resuscitator which forces oxygen into the lungs. The monitor line jumped and paused as before, but this time, when the beats came back, they came back more regularly and evenly spaced.

I pushed the button on the valve to press air into the man. His chest heaved heavily. Thinking that I needed to lessen the pressure with the next blast, I waited a moment. To my surprise, the valve of the resuscitator tripped on its own. The man had started his own breathing!

The other fireman was working with Drew, setting up his IV. Drew got it first try and administered an ampoule of 50 cc's of sodium bicarbonate, which counteracts the lactic acid build up during periods of breathlessness. Lactic acid chemically short-circuits the heart, causing it to get irritable was the belief at the time.

The woman was talking with someone on the other side of the door, on the stoop. Two more volunteer firemen brushed past, lugging in our gurney; another two behind them. A County Sheriff followed. Now there were six volunteer firemen and a cop in the house, then another cop, followed by someone I didn't know. Apparently, half the town of Orcutt had been as bored as we had been!

The man began taking about every fifth breath on his own. I handed the pressure valve to one of the firemen and made radio contact with the hospital. The firemen and Drew carefully put the man on the gurney and then moved him past his wife and out the door. She looked down at him as he passed, and then up to Drew.

"So," she asked, "he's breathing, and you're taking him to hospital now?"

"That's right," Drew replied, "he'll be at Marian."

She leaned around to the man on the other side of the door. "I'm sorry for your trouble," she said. "My daughter was wrong. I guess you can go now."

After I contacted the doctor and filled him in, I went outside.

This had been everybody's big deal. Not only was there the fire rescue truck, but a fire engine, two police cars, two civilian cars, and right alongside our ambulance, a hearse. Putting it all together, I realized the man to whom the woman had been talking was from the funeral home. He was now getting back in to his vehicle. We beat him, by God, I thought. We beat him!

By the time we got him to the hospital, the man was still unconscious but taking every third breath himself. His color improved considerably. He was still cold to the touch, but then again, so were we.

We went to bed early that night and slept right through to the end of our shift at eight a.m. the next morning. We arose, returned the blankets we borrowed from the ambulance, went through shift-change rigmarole with the oncoming crew and then hopped into Drew's car to take a quick trip to the hospital before we went home. Drew had his eye on a nurse working in Intensive Care that day and I was always looking.

In the nurse's station outside the cubicle that housed our only call on that 72 hour shift; our patient's doctor came in.

"It was the strangest thing," Doctor Edelman ran his fingers through his silver hair, unusually long for a doctor of his age, "his wife called me, told me he was dead, and then hung right up. I figured I better call for you guys."

"Then she called her daughter," Drew offered, "and *she* just picked up the phone and called the funeral home."

"Kind of lucky we were right there," I said. "If the hearse had made it first, it might have cooked his goose. We coulda had a big ol' fight for the body; just like the old days!"

"You're probably right," said the doctor. "I hadn't even gotten off the phone with the dispatcher, and she told me you were right there. How did you manage that?"

"Oh, come on now, Doc," Drew picked up the slack, and I was glad, "you know as well as we do, when someone isn't meant to go..."

Dr. Edelman raised his hand in a "hold on" motion. Drew trailed off, waiting. The doc looked as if he were searching for words.

"Yeah," the doctor said, finally, "God screws around with everything to make schmucks like us look like heroes."

He said it very matter-of-factly and without a hint of derision, yet there was a solemnity to it that made me wonder what devils he had been grappling with lately.

"Well," the doctor went on, "he was asking for you guys. May as well see what kind of reward he has for you."

Reward? Now that was a switch! Up to that point in my career, I had been *thanked* by a patient whom I saved once. Reward wasn't even in my vocabulary. Not because I didn't think I deserved or earned it now and then, but because it just didn't happen. Drew was smiling at my reaction; he winked and crooked his head toward the man's cubicle.

"Let's do it," he said.

We could hear the man's raspy cough. Drew pulled the curtain aside, and we stood in front of him. I wondered if we were both waiting for him to recognize us, jump out of bed and give us a hug.

To our confusion, the man looked at us with the disdain that is usually reserved for the waitress who grabs your beer bottle before you've finished it. Drew and I looked at each other and kind of giggled.

"Um," I said, "We're the paramedics that were at your house last night. We brought you here."

He looked at us and then gave us what I thought might have been the start of a smile, but was only the precursor to a cough. The man started to speak in a crackly voice, but then coughed again. He motioned us to come closer. Like a couple of love-starved puppy dogs, we moved in ridiculously close to him. Neither of us wanted to miss this. Moments like this were enough to keep you going for months.

When you're pulling someone out of Death's grasp, it's all about the moment and the task at hand. Encountering that person again afterwards, it's a whole different story. When you first met, he was dead. Now he's alive, and what has he come back to tell you?

"My...my...," the man stammered. We both leaned forward and placed our heads just a few inches from his mouth so we could hear.

"My wallet," was what he finally said.

Drew and I stood up straight and looked at each other. He wants his wallet? Uh-oh, I thought, I hate this. I'm not there for tips. The doc said "reward" and the last of the last things I'd expect is money! I started to form the words in my head that would allow me to respectfully, diplomatically decline.

"My wallet," he said again after clearing his throat. He raised his voice, and, with firmness, concluded his sentence, "I want it back!"

We still weren't sure what was going on. He coughed, cleared his throat, and now, with a touch of menace, made himself clear.

"Someone took my wallet," he said with as much forcefulness as he could muster. "You better give it back."

Drew and I looked at the old codger. Drew gave him a crooked smile, and I realized I was doing the same. Without saying a word to the man or each other, we turned and walked out of the cubicle, out of the ICU, out of the hospital, got into Drew's car and left that shift behind us.

Chapter Three
MOMENTS

Out of the corner of my eye, I could see the man rolling his eyes up toward me. He asked, "Mommy?"

This was not the first time that such a thing had happened to me during a call. Usually, it occurred during delirium. This time, though, the man was very lucid.

My mouth knew what to do. It said, "What was that, John?"

The strapping man, neck broken, wrapped from his waist to the top of his skull in a rigidly supportive nylon-covered splint immobilizing his head, neck and spine replied, "S...sorry."

Perhaps five adults had said words just like that to me over the course of my career. The words came spontaneously and totally out of context, from a very deep place; a place full of fear and total dependence where the child within cries out for help.

My eyes were telling my hands what to do with the numerous tubes, lines, Velcro® strips, cardiac monitor electrodes and bandages wrapped around and slung over John's wife, lying unconscious on the ambulance's gurney, about a foot and a half across the aisle from him.

"I want to touch Kathy." He said rolling his eyes toward me. "Can I touch Kathy? I guess I can't."

He answered his own question. I noticed my hand leaving the ambulance's inboard oxygen outlet. It had obviously just reconnected the oxygen tubing that went to Kathy's nose. I didn't even remember seeing it was disconnected. The hand just took care of it.

"John," I said, "we're gonna be at the hospital soon. I'm taking good care of Kathy."

Am I? I thought. Somebody was, but it didn't seem like me. I was not even there. I was just a very intense...presence? All I knew was in this moment, I was a bump away from losing two patients, and I didn't want that to happen. There was nothing but the lives of those patients.

There were a million things to do. Recheck Kathy's blood pressure, and then check John's. Listen to Kathy's lungs, and then run a pin up and down John's arm to re-check his level of sensation. Make sure there was enough air pressure in Kathy's M.A.S.T. (Military Anti-Shock Trousers) and say a word to John to make sure he was still with me. Check the cardiac monitor on Kathy, then call in to the hospital and give them an update. Listen to Kathy's lungs again, and with the stethoscope still in my ears, double-check John's blood pressure.

All the time expecting at any second for Kathy to stop breathing and go into cardiac arrest and for John to lose consciousness, and then, with his own blood pressure plummeting, die as well.

Back and forth, back and forth...First to the unconscious young woman, who had been impaled, had a crushed abdomen and chest, a head injury, and whose only link to life was a prayer. And then to her husband whose neck had been broken so badly a millimeter of motion in the wrong direction could instantly send him into oblivion.

But everything was getting done. I was alone in the back of the ambulance with them, yet everything was getting done. All was happening; without a thought. Eyes would see, hands would do; ears would hear, mouth would speak; hands would feel, eyes would check: On and on as if absolutely nothing was going through my brain.

I was eyes, ears and hands and just a feeling in the center of my chest of pure internal silence. Suspended in time and moving in a vacuum, I didn't have a name or a job; I was movement choreographed by something much greater than myself.

A string of relentless moments brought me to this state of being.

The day, beginning about 20 hours earlier, had started out typically. At 8:00 a.m. my shift started. Two routine transfers before lunch, a quick push of glucose into a diabetic's vein around 2:00 p.m., and then, at around 4:00, my partner, Jim, and I brought one of the morning's patients back to the nursing home from the hospital. Routine as they come.

Then, we got the "LD to LA" — a long distance transfer to Los Angeles, about 200 miles south. It was a non-emergency transfer of an elderly woman to the Doheny Eye Institute for surgery. The call was timed so we'd leave Santa Maria 4:45 p.m., hit a rush-hour surge in Santa Barbara an hour later, wade through the tail end of Ventura's rush-hour, and then set a slow but steady pace through the San Fernando Valley and on to L.A., reaching our destination by about eight that night.

With some summer light left to get us through L.A. and the valley again, we expected to have smooth sailing home. It would be a total round trip of about

Moments in the Death of a Flesh Mechanic...a healer's rebirth

six and a half hours. Then, I projected; we'd be asleep by about eleven; a full day, but tolerable.

Both Jim and I enjoyed LDs. Jim was a local boy who had the wanderlust. He just loved to drive. That's why, he told me, he became an EMT, "I got the driving crazies," he said.

Movement was my passion. I enjoyed the feeling of miles passing. I had abandoned my car for a motorcycle long ago, and any time I could arrange a few days off, I'd go touring somewhere; anywhere.

Movement provided a backbeat for whatever I was doing. On LDs with alert patients, it was fun, like a social call to talk of times I'd never seen. With the grumps or lethargic not requiring care, reading a book was fine. In critical cases, each second was accounted for.

Arriving earlier than planned, the trip had gone uneventfully until about 7:30, upon our return. The sun was a maroon, basketball-sized orb through the smog to our left as we headed north. It hovered about 30 degrees above the horizon, leaving us about a half hour of light. We were in a bottleneck of traffic, moving at about a steady 50 miles per hour, surprisingly slow for that time of day.

As we crested a hill, we saw about a half mile ahead of us five perfectly clear lanes of traffic. There was an odd, out-of-place clot of cars that we had to get through first, though. Sometimes, you'd think in terms of "Let's check this out; it might be an emergency." On this night, we were thinking, "Let's get through this crap and get home to bed!"

Being in an ambulance has its distinct advantages. In a private car, you can dog a slow-moving vehicle for miles before it gets the hint to speed up or get out of the way. The sight of an ambulance moving aggressively toward you in your mirror — even without its lights or siren on — prompts a response. Sometimes, it spells trouble!

Jim used our imposing form to advantage. Within two minutes, we were at the head of the pack. What we saw astounded us!

There was a car in the number three lane traveling about 50 miles an hour. It was proceeding just ahead of two cars to either side of it, like the vanguard of a V-shaped flight formation. Initially, we wondered aloud if there wasn't some sort of game being played. There was, but not by anything human or made by humans.

A lone, dusky gray and black pigeon appeared from the right of the lead car. Flying to three feet above it, it flapped its wings furiously and overtook the vehicle. Then, dropping down and back to the car on the lead car's left, it swooped low and into a space just about a foot behind the side-view mirror of the car and actually started drafting it!

That car then sped up to 55 and took the lead. The pigeon casually flapped its wings and, locked into the momentum, paced the car inches from its side window. Then, as if fired by a slingshot, it flew above and ahead of the car. It tipped its wings and slid back behind the side-view mirror of the car from which it first materialized.

We took our position on the left wing of the formation and, fascinated, moved with the procession of fellow gapers for about three miles. The pigeon was going back and forth from the first car to the second, drafting, sling-shooting ahead, dropping back and drafting again.

It never came to us, although we were beckoning to it to do so. We figured a pigeon that cool could understand our ridiculous gestures!

Jim and I came to the conclusion that of all the pigeons in world history, this one found the perfect circumstances to propel it at speeds never before attained by any of its species. "This is one dedicated freeway flyer," Jim said.

Just at the same time as we emerged from under a series of three overpass bridges, the pigeon, as quickly as it appeared, swung high, fell back and vanished into thin air. Jim kept checking the rear-view mirror to see if the traffic pattern would repeat. It did not.

Then, our temperature light went on. We pulled off at the next exit and had to drive a few blocks before we found an open gas station. When we stopped, the vehicle was steaming.

We located a pinhole leak in a heater hose. The man on duty barely spoke English, nor was there a mechanic. After hosing down the engine and replenishing the water, we went to a nearby 7-Eleven®, bought a two-and-a-half-gallon container of drinking water and took off. Our intention was to get out of "Smell A." and then stop for dinner. So much for intentions; now, we had to get the rig home before it blew up!

This was not terribly uncommon. Typically, private ambulance firms were always behind on the maintenance of their vehicles. That led to breakdowns like this, usually of a minor variety, but while pushing the vehicle in an emergency it could compound the situation considerably.

Every half hour, whether we needed it or not, we pulled off the freeway, found a gas station, replenished the water and proceeded. It is mostly downhill or flat from the tail end of Thousand Oaks to Gaviota Pass — over 100 miles, so strain on the engine was minimal. The sun had dropped, and by now, it was turning into a typically cool Southern California night. Luck was with us, we thought. Perhaps we were being saved for better things. Food didn't even seem as important now as sleep.

At the top of Refugio Grade, a steep rise going from sea level to about 1500 feet just on the other side of a tunnel that bores through the Santa Ynez Mountains, steam started to spray from under the hood. We pulled over, inspected the engine to see the pinhole was no longer a pin hole, dumped some

Moments in the Death of a Flesh Mechanic...a healer's rebirth

water in and coasted downhill until we cooled and then went on to Buellton. Fifteen minutes was now our range. We made three more stops before we traded ambulances in Santa Maria.

By the time we kicked off our boots, not even bothering to take our clothes off, and lay down in our beds at Marian Hospital quarters it was midnight. Not bad, only an hour behind schedule. Before I nodded out, I realized my partner and I hadn't spoken to each other for an hour.

At 12:20 a.m., our pager tone went off. We silently put our boots back on, staggered out to the unit, got in and went to the call, only about a minute away. When we got on the scene — prophetically, the Black Eye Bar — police officers asked us to examine a couple of drunks who had been fighting in the street. The officers wanted us to give them medical clearance before they threw them into jail.

Just a basic exam was all that was necessary. With violent drunks, it's much wiser to do an exam with your eyes only if you can get away with it until you know you're safe. That's what I did. Jim, on the other hand, undertook a complete hands-on, head-to-toe evaluation of his patient. That was good, I thought. He's taking practice seriously.

I'd like to say my own lack of action had been intuition, but I remember admitting to myself I was feeling lazy and the hell with the drunks. My visual exam at a distance of about two feet from the larger, smellier and bloodier of the pair prompted me to instinctively back up. Sure enough, a powerful four foot trail of vomited dinner exploded from his mouth. Pizza and beer were my new thoughts as a part of the stream hit me; and projectile vomiting and possible head injury, too.

"How's yours?" I asked Jim as I brushed chunks off my shirt.

"He's okay," he replied.

"Let's get this guy in," I said. "Too close to the hospital to call in for orders. You attend. Just protect his airway."

"His airway and my shirt," Jim said; "Gotcha!"

Jim was happy. He liked responsibility being thrust on him. He snapped our gurney out of the back of the rig like a pro and set it alongside the drunk, who was mumbling incoherently to himself. We raised him into the back and took off for the hospital. Within eight minutes of our arrival on the scene, the drunk was being examined by the doctor in the Emergency Room.

We finished basic paperwork. It was 1:00 a.m. and we were back in our room. I put my uniform in a bag, got into my jump suit, then took the bag out to the end of the hallway, opened the exit door and tossed it outside by the wall. It would be there in the morning.

Five after one, and I was sound asleep. One-fifteen, the tone went off again. Before I heard the words come through the speaker, my boots were on, and I was out the door. I realized I'd better check on Jim.

Going back into the room, I shook him. He was still very sound asleep. Another shake and when I was sure he was awake, I went out to the unit, sat in the passenger seat and called in to Dispatch.

"Medic Eight is 10-8 and ready to copy," I said.

"Medic Eight..." came back the dispatcher, "disregard. Police Department canceled their request for assistance."

"Uh-huh," I said and put the microphone back on its clip.

Jim was just coming out of the door of the hospital. I hooked my arm in his and turned him around. "Back to bed, it's a Bogey!"

At 1:20, Jim was asleep again; his boots still on his feet. I lay awake, tossing and turning and unsuccessfully groping for sleep for about 10 minutes when the tone went off again.

This time, Jim jumped up out of bed and out the door. I found myself running to catch up. He hopped right into the driver's seat and looked over toward the passenger door. He did a double-take when he saw that I wasn't already sitting in the seat, but just getting into the cab.

"Uh...you drop something?" he asked, slightly confused.

"Nuh-uh," I answered.

"I'm sorry, man," he apologized, trying to shake the sleep away. "I didn't even hear that tone. Thanks for waking me."

I didn't bother to tell him that that had been one whole call ago!

"Medic Eight," called dispatch, "report of a heart attack at 675 North Broadway respond Code Three; Medic Seven, move to cover."

"Eight copys," I said into the mic, "Code Three."

In a flash, we were there. Jim's adrenaline was pumping. I was marginal at best.

Trudging to the top of the second story of the home, I found I still had to lug my equipment another 10 steps up a narrow staircase to the tiny attic of the old house. When I realized what was going on in that makeshift room, I began carefully putting down my equipment, moaning "Wonderful!" to myself.

This patient fell out and down into the most inaccessible part of that room, a foot-wide swath of space between a double bed that took up most of the room and a wall. The man was large, and he was crammed into the tiny little crawlspace, and he had a lot of damned nerve!

Moments in the Death of a Flesh Mechanic...a healer's rebirth

His son and daughter-in-law, in their bedroom below, heard him hit the floor. It had only been just a few minutes earlier. The man was in his late 50s. He had no prior history of significant medical problems. There was no avoiding this one, even though all I really wanted to do was go back to sleep.

If you're a paramedic long enough, you'll find yourself doing anything. Critical decisions, like who to work up and who not, will be based on maintaining one's ability to function. Sometimes, it comes to saving yourself to be able to get to the next patient, or five patients; or maybe it could be because you need that last scrap of strength to keep your marriage together. There's trial and error, and lingering doubt.

You wonder, "Was that guy salvageable, or was I just too fucking lazy?" The more experience you get, you see how people who have no chance to come back, come back. So, over time, it's fair to say, it gets even more difficult to make a final call. You just never know. It boils down to learning what you are personally capable of living with.

This harsh reality lives most vividly in high-volume call areas, usually big cities. There, the medics make judgment calls quickly — sometimes too quickly — just so they can be available for...

Jim leaped over the bed and began CPR while I started to open my equipment boxes and get ready. The Fire Department arrived and I had to move my boxes down to the second floor. They disassembled the bed and passed it down the stairs so we could get to the patient. Once the bed was down, I retrieved my boxes and handed anybody who could do anything pieces of equipment and asked each to get ready to hand them back to me when I asked; like a surgeon setting up his scrub nurses.

I found myself methodically doing a mental check list to prevent myself from forgetting anything. I was struggling to keep my mind in the situation. Syringes, laryngoscope, endotracheal tubes, tape, cardiac monitor/defibrillator, K-Y® jelly, pads, oxygen, oh shit, pediatric drip, not regular, 18 gauge needle, not the 14; dammit, get it together!

Before long, each of the four firemen had something in his hand. During that time, working with the Santa Maria Fire Department was a pleasure. They worked work well with the local medics and were extremely fastidious when it came to handling medical situations on their own. Sad to say, this was not always true with other county departments.

The room was clear, the patient flat on his back in the center of the floor. Jim continued CPR, while I began therapy. Each action began with an observation translated into a thought, and then followed with moving the appropriate body part. Each sequence had to be pushed through my exhaustion. It was a step-by-step process with control and forced consciousness being the drivers of my rhythm.

Once I completed intubating him, I started to build energy and move more smoothly; my second wind came through. I moved into my Mechanic mode. Seeing the need for a specific piece of equipment, I'd remember who had what, turn to the person and ask for it.

Defibrillation was followed by placing an IV line, administering sodium bicarbonate, then epinephrine, then a second defibrillation with successful conversion followed by atropine to speed the heart rate and, boom; a good pulse. Textbook! The words even came to me as I completed each phase. "Defibrillate. No good. Go for IV. Good hit! Bicarb. Epi. Hit again. Four-hundred now. Good! Nope, too slow. No pulse yet. Okay, call in for atropine. Thank you, Doc, and *Bingo*!"

My mind was clear and my consciousness was in control. By the time one of the firemen called out, "We've got a blood pressure of 90 over 64!" I was feeling pretty satisfied — like the hub of a wheel that everything had depended on to make the wagon move.

With six of us to handle the now stable patient, it was easy to get him strapped on to a "flat" and down the flights of stairs to the gurney and into the ambulance. Funny, I thought. It all came easy; to *me*!

By the time we got to the hospital, the patient was dead.

It was now 3:00 a.m. and I was in the emergency room on the phone getting our times for our records. Our companion ambulance, Medic Seven, had gotten a call while it was moved up to cover our area. I was just about ready to let my exhaustion set in.

The dispatcher put me on hold while she took another call. I prayed it wasn't about us. I couldn't even stomach the idea of going on move-up, nodding and then having to drag my bones back to the base.

"I'm sorry about this," she said, "but we need you to head out to downtown Los Alamos for a possible car accident."

"We're Code Three," I said.

Then, I grabbed Jim, who was cleaning up equipment. We shoved everything into our drug box, hopped into the rig and took off.

"It's three o'clock in the morning," Jim said. "How could anything be going on in Los Alamos? Nothing ever happens there at three o'clock in the afternoon, for Gods sakes; Ever!"

Too tired to answer, all I wanted to do was sleep. But I had to keep awake and push into fuller wakefulness. It was crucial now, because my partner, whose well-being I depended on, was as tired as I; and he was driving! I opened my window and was blasted by the chilly air. We had the emergency lights on, but no siren. We shot on to the highway and hit 90 miles per hour for the 18-mile trip to Los Alamos.

Moments in the Death of a Flesh Mechanic...a healer's rebirth

"You're right." I forced myself to engage in the conversation, "Nothin' there except antique stores and that bed-and-breakfast place..."

"Love that town," Jim said. "You know, they're finishing with that Victorian house next door to...it's the Union *Hotel* not a B and B."

"Fine, whatever," I said. "The plan is to make the whole town like that; like you're stepping back into time. An Old West town..."

"Authentic," Jim interrupted. "Every bit of wood to build the hotel, the Victorian, and the sidewalk was pulled from 1880's barns!"

"They plan on keeping that up, too," I replied.

Suddenly, Jim stopped picking up the threads of small talk; he was turning his full concentration to the road. 12 minutes later, while I jabbered away incessantly for both of us, we drove up the deserted main street of Los Alamos. We passed an old travel trailer on blocks on the left of the road. There was a dent where the side and bottom of the trailer articulated, just above the blocks which had been jilted but not knocked out. The last quarter of the dent had a shard of metal sticking out of it.

From the point of impact were four skid marks that lead to a 1960s vintage Shelby Mustang at a 30 degree angle to the road. Its right, engine side was wrapped around a telephone pole a few yards away from the Union Hotel. There were a few V-shaped gouges in its driver's side, running from just behind the headlight, midway into the door.

Coming from the other direction through the steam billowing out from under the damaged car's hood, which wasn't crumpled so much as splintered, another car skid to a halt in front of it.

Jim pulled the ambulance behind the crashed vehicle at an angle, protecting it and the other car from traffic to the rear. I flicked on the white side lights of the ambulance to illuminate the scene. I could see the car was made of fiberglass-like stuff. The driver's side was shredded into strips and shards that intertwined with the car's metal framework.

A man jumped out of the newly arrived vehicle. On his belt, was a police-band scanner. Four red lights on it flashed in sequence as it picked up transmissions from vital protection agencies.

"It's all right," he almost screamed out to us. "I'm a Vollie!"

Vollie, what? I thought. Any help was good help, even a Hot Dog, I decided. As he sidled up to the crashed vehicle, I told Jim to follow me and quickly jumped out of the ambulance and went to the passenger's door, which was closest to me.

Triage, the evaluation of the situation and sorting of patients according to severity, always comes first. Our target was the car. This, night, it would have been no surprise to find ten people crammed into it!

There is nothing more harrowing then triage. When you're first on scene, you must review the whole situation. Even if others are there, calmly and methodically, you and your partner must go from vehicle to vehicle, person to person, and set priorities. You're in charge and the most important role you can play is to direct the actions of the medics who follow you in. You're not so much a medic as a coordinator.

You can open the victims' airways as you go. Maybe wrap a tourniquet around a limb real quick, but there's not time to take to stop someone's bleeding from anywhere else. In that period you could lose two more who were salvageable. If you left one car to go to another and by the time you came back to the first car a person was dead, well, then, there was nothing you could have done anyway.

Once everyone has been assessed for severity, you set priorities. Under normal circumstances, you'd have a chance to save one or two borderline cases. In multiple victim accidents, however, they must wait for a back-up ambulance or more help. An open chest injury, as example, where blood is being lost and there is lung involvement would, with two paramedics, have a chance. But in a multiple situation, even if the patient is alert and conscious, your time is better spent on a patient with a fracture and severed artery and maybe another with an amputation. In the meantime, the chest-injury patient drowns in his own fluids.

My most vivid nightmare around this work was that very scenario. Finding myself amidst a multiple-multiple car wreck, I, without a partner of course, went from car to car. In the first I found a teenager with chest injuries as described. Leaving him alone with his vocal and haunting agony, I turned to the next car; same situation, but a girl now. One after another, through five vehicles I had to turn from the desperate gasps of a teenager only to walk into the death throes of another!

The harrowing thing about triage is, in the worst case scenario, you're literally choosing who will live and who will die. It's your decision, and, in reality, you never know; you can only play the odds.

As soon as we started to look into the passenger window with a flashlight to examine the patients, I heard this:

"What the fuck're you guys doin'? What kind a medics are you, anyway? Wanna get in the car, you get in the Goddamn car!"

I heard a grunt. The man was grabbing pieces of the car's side panel helter-skelter to get closer to the driver's door. My flashlight lit the interior of the car. In the passenger seat was a young man, seemingly intact and leaning against the back of his seat, but my eyes went directly to the driver — a young woman covered in blood and moaning in pain.

Embedded in her left side, below her rib cage, was a two-inch-wide strip of fiberglass that had shred from the ripped door into her.

Moments in the Death of a Flesh Mechanic...a healer's rebirth

"God, please, NO!" I screamed, but it was too late.

I heard an, "Unhh!" and watched as eight inches of that rogue slice of the car came sliding out of the woman's side. Blood oozed out of the hole it left. The bearded face of a half-drunk man wearing a baseball cap peeked in at me through the window with a proud, cocky smile.

"Almost there!" he beamed. It all took place in an instant.

The next thing I knew, Jim was on the other side of the car, had already pushed the drunk away and was putting his hand, wrapped in a bandage, on the wound and pressing.

And that's where I lost me.

Hundreds of things happened. The police arrived. They made sure there were no other victims. They got that miserable helper out of there. More passersby arrived. We had to have had a lot of help because somehow, that young couple got splinted, pulled out of that coffin of a car, and then loaded into the back of the ambulance.

It wasn't until the moment my patient called out "Mommy" that I awakened. During all the previous moments, it was like there was no "me" there at all — no "me" to hold on to. In my exhaustion and terror and despair and rage, I had ceased to be. A big chunk of time vanished from my life. At the same time, something wondrous had happened.

When I helplessly witnessed that strip of fiberglass sliding out of the woman's side, I was consumed by powerlessness. In cases of impalement, the only thing that keeps the patient alive is keeping the invading object in place so it "plugs" the wound and keeps the loss of blood to a minimum. Once the object is removed, the dam bursts.

If the plunging feeling in my belly had words, they would have been these: "I'm the medic dammit; it's all supposed to revolve around me! This can't happen; *I'm* here!" But it did, and I was helpless. So, in that moment, I gave up. In my mind's eye, I threw up my hands and said, "That's it, God...this baby is *yours*!" And the moment I got out of the way was the moment that things really started to happen. At the time it felt like I wasn't even there to witness it.

John's call for Mommy snapped me back. My body was doing things to manage my patients, but by then, it was maintenance. The hard part had already passed. It was as if each of my body parts was on its own volition and then someone said, "Wake up! You're one person!"

Jim was now driving us to the hospital, carefully monitoring the unit's speed so its movement was minimal. In back of the ambulance, there was an atmospheric lull, like being in the eye of a hurricane.

My body continued to go through the movements necessary to keep that couple alive. At the same time, flashes of memory came back to me, filling me in on what had transpired during the time I had ceased to be. With each memory came a feeling that was accompanied by the flash of a scene. And all were linked to something in the present.

It has taken me many years to be able to unravel, sort through and then find the words to describe my experience in those moments.

The passenger, John, knew he was helpless. His words betrayed him even though he was working very hard to appear everything was all right. From the start, he almost had me fooled, too. On first contact with the hapless couple, when Jim went to Kathy, my hands just went into action to begin an assessment on John. That was their job, and they knew it. John was awake and alert; even smiling.

"My name's Russ." I said, "I'm a paramedic. Is there anybody else besides you two?"

In the bucket seat of the Mustang, John's head was tilted back, lying on the adjustable head rest in its lowermost position. John was tall, and his head was barely balanced on it.

"Nope, just us" he said, keeping his eyes fixed on the roof as casually as if he was looking through a sunroof. Only problem was, there wasn't a sunroof! He was too damn lucid after a wreck like that, too.

"But I can't seem to move very well," he said matter-of-factly and with no alarm whatsoever.

I started from the top of his head, feeling for injury. Finding no more than a few minor bruises, I slipped my hand behind his neck to gently palpate. It was like mush!

"Can you feel this?" I asked him and pinched the skin over his collarbone hard. It was no surprise to me when he replied, "Feel what?"

So there it was; a broken neck. Extensive swelling had begun. Amidst it, it was hard to tell where the fracture was located. A few quick questions and pinches told me that he was totally unable to feel any part of his body besides the skin on his face.

The spinal cord begins at the base of the medulla oblongata, the lowermost portion of the brain, which controls automatic function such as respiration and heartbeat. It's the most basic part of our brains; often called the "Lizard Brain". Once swelling begins, and pressure encroaches on that vital center, it's all over. So in that moment, after the incident with his wife, I knew that he, too, was a hairsbreadth away from death. Whatever illusion I had of control evaporated into the void.

Finishing my complete head-to-toe exam of John, I found no other apparent injuries. Yet, with his inability to feel anything, I knew I may have missed something; maybe many things. I had to stop my probing and force myself to move on.

Moments in the Death of a Flesh Mechanic...a healer's rebirth

A Sheriff's officer came up to me. I placed his hands in mine and carefully wrapped them around John's jawbone and sides of his head and locked them into place around him as support.

"Whatever you do," I told the sheriff, "don't move him."

The officer had the same look on his face you get when you are asked to hold an infant for the first time. You're told, "Be real careful with the head. The neck's weak; you have to support it, or it will flop around and damage the baby." Please, I prayed, don't damage the baby.

An infant's head; helpless, and me at the scene; powerless.

Now, back in the unit, right after John had mistaken me for his mother, it hit me that, indeed, John was as an infant, totally dependent on me and one mistake away from death.

I would have liked to have been the one who could have made a difference, but I knew that it was out of my hands. I was simply a mechanic who, somewhere along the line had been handed a sacred trust. So when John looked up at me with those imploring eyes, I felt embarrassed. At that point, I knew there were a hundred simple things that I could purposefully or inadvertently do to hasten his death, but I couldn't think of one thing that I could do to preserve his life.

Prevent his movement? Maybe. But control the motion of the ambulance, or the degree to which his blood flooded his injury, or delay his crucial spinal nerves from short-circuiting? No. It was out of my hands. I wanted to direct his energy to that which truly was in charge. But that would tip him off and lose me whatever illusion of control I was trying to convey I had. He knew he was helpless, but he didn't have a clue how close to death he really was. John was still very lucid. All he thought was wrong was that he couldn't move.

What could I say? "John, better start praying because it's all up to God now." No, in this culture, those are not words of reassurance. He would pray if that was his inclination. My role was to look and act as if I was in control. So I acted as if I was. Underneath it all, the last items in my bag of tricks were my own prayers, and I was using them big time!

Switching over to work on Kathy, his wife, a different set of memories and feelings welled up in me.

Kathy had no cognitive thought to stand between her and her Creator. I imagined her sitting at His/Her feet, waiting. Once again, with the choices I might have been able to make on her behalf, with the actions I could either take deliberately or inadvertently I could possibly stumble and tip the scales to save her life. Then again, one mistake and... But what distinguished her from John was I sensed in this very moment, she was working things out *directly* with her Creator.

Perhaps it was this impression that prompted me to leave my own conscious thought behind and simply allow something else to move through me. It wasn't as if I had a choice. It was just happening. I was consumed by the experience. I felt as if *I* were being moved.

I couldn't handle the awesome responsibility on my own. This situation would demand hyper vigilance and extreme amounts of control, but in my exhaustion and despair and frustration, I had lost the capability to do anything but "be", as if my head had fallen off. A casual observer may have looked and said, "Now there's a paramedic in charge!", but that wasn't the case. I was as out of control as my patients, but my body, still able, seemed to be following something else's directions.

When I left John — literally in the hands of the Officer — and crossed over to Jim as he supported Kathy in his arms, I was surprised to see the driver's door was open.

Miraculously, the car must have ricocheted off the trailer and responded to hitting the pole in such a way as not to have damaged the door's locking mechanism. Of course, it was a miracle. For me, it was just a new piece of information. I was not surprised by anything.

"His neck is snapped," I said, pointing to the passenger. "The cop's holding him stable for now. What's going on here?"

I looked closely at Kathy's eyes. They had changed. When I first shined my flashlight on her, there was a very pained look in her eyes matched with moaning. Now, everything was different.

There are degrees of spark in an injured person's eyes that indicate just how far gone he or she is. There is no textbook that explains it. It is something that can only be felt through your eyes.

As a person nears death, the spark does not get dim or weaken. It gets distant — as if something deep inside is going away. There's no other way to describe it. In Kathy's case, when I looked back into her eyes again, I saw that her spark had jumped way back. She was not conscious enough to be aware, yet not distant enough to be gone. The largest part of her was sitting in Limbo, barely in sight.

"She's unconscious now," Jim started as he gave me his full evaluation of the woman: "Pulse 110 and thready; B.P. 80/60; respirations; 18. Left side closed head injury. There's a dent about two centimeters deep just behind the temple above her ear. Jaw and mouth are okay. Shoulder girdle okay. Arms clear except for bruises. Left side ribs probable multiple fractures. Noisy left lung. Wet. Looks like she hit the steering wheel at an angle, then bounced her head off the window support. There's a two-inch entry wound — incision — just below lower ribs left side. External bleeding is under control. No exit wound visible. Abdomen hard on left side on palpation. Crepitus in her left pelvis and hip. Negative for fractures in her lower left extremities. Right side absent of injuries across the board. No evidence of spinal fracture."

Jesus, what a good job he did, I thought! Someone rolled the gurney over with our equipment on it. Jim must have directed that also.

Jim was doing really well. But he was still my EMT, my assistant. I was accountable to use him properly. At that time, I was hard pressed to trust anyone with my patients. After what happened at the car, the sheriff was the biggest gamble I was willing to take outside of my partner. Even at that, every cell of my body cried out, "Caution!"

"Don't leave my side," I told Jim evenly, "unless I tell you."

"Gotcha," Jim said.

Part of me had become fiercely protective of my patients. It understood the role it was meant to play in this drama and, moving on its own instincts, would not let anyone else move except by its command. Not even me.

Unless Kathy was stabilized immediately, it would be all over. Jim and I carefully slid the woman out the door, to a long wooden backboard and on to the gurney. Then, we put her into the M.A.S.T. – Velcro®-secured inflatable trousers that, when expanded, auto-transfuse blood from the lower extremities up to the vital organs to stave off shock.

I took care not to inflate the compartment around her abdomen to avoid putting pressure on her injuries. Now, there was little external bleeding. That could have meant one or both of two things: Either blood flow had been cut off, or she was bleeding into her abdominal cavity.

Jim turned to setting up my IV lines while I took her blood pressure again. I could not hear the sounds; I could only feel pulsations with my fingers on the main artery inside the bend of her elbow. Her BP was 60 by palpation now; low wasn't the word!

I started two IVs, one in each of her arms, with the largest bore needles I had, 12 gauge; large enough for someone to breathe through. After the IVs were in place, I raised the angle of the backboard to elevate her head slightly to compensate for her head injury. I covered her with blankets. I opened her eyes and looked into them with my penlight.

Technically, I was checking her pupils. Realistically, I was looking for her spark. That something was drifting further away. Something not only vital to her, but in some way that I couldn't grasp, vital to me. I found myself tenderly touching her cheek with my fingers. I had to let her know she had some connection to the living even as I sensed the deepest part of her was surrendering to the will of *her* God.

The next few moves happened like clockwork. I had nothing to do with them. Jim took the girl on the gurney to the ambulance while I crossed to the passenger side. I replaced the officer's hands with mine as Jim got help lifting the gurney into the back of the rig. The officer took position with Kathy while Jim hooked her up to the inboard oxygen and the cardiac monitor. Jim went and then grabbed the flat stretcher and short backboard splint. He then came back to me.

Jim worked around me as I guided John into proper, supported position for application of the splint, which meant keeping his head in the exact position we had found it. Within five minutes, John and that splint were one, and we laid him out on the flat stretcher and carried him into the ambulance. One hundred fifty things could have gone wrong in those moments — each with fatal results — but nothing did.

On board, Kathy's blood pressure was hovering right at about 80 by palpation; this after flooding her with 2,000 c.c.s of fluid. John's blood pressure was dropping, so I started an IV on him also. And then another, just in case. Once the IVs were in place, I instructed Jim to "Get us home!" and got to work with the next phase.

It was as if everything I had ever heard in the classroom, or seen on every call, or every mistake I had ever made and every corrective action I had ever taken in my experience as a medic was being surgically applied for the benefit of these strangers. And then, there were those actions I was taking and decisions I was making that seemed to come out of the experience of lives that I had never lived, calls I had never been on, and from connections I had never come close to making.

When John called out "Mommy," my focus was on Kathy. When I was through with that most recent burst of activity, I turned back to John and saw his eyes were closed.

My first thought was to panic and do something fast to bring him back. But I knew much good had been accomplished in the last few minutes by not doing anything that came from my thoughts. My head was screaming out to me: "He's dying, he's giving up, don't let him fall out. If he falls out, he's dead, bring him back. Bring him BACK; hurry!" Instead, I bypassed it all and, taking in a deep breath, went to someplace deep within my chest, a place surprisingly calm and absent of fear.

Once again, my body started to move. My head calmly leaned over and I put my cheek just above John's nose and mouth to check his breathing. It was irregular but sufficient. My hands boosted the oxygen to six liters from four, then my right hand took his pulse (eighty), and my mouth whispered "John?" in his ear. Then my eyes watched.

He opened his eyes. They were clear. The spark was there, fully present, yet distant. His eyes held something I had just seen in Kathy's. John, too, was surrendering, but in a different way. He looked up at the ceiling and said, "Tired," and then toward me for reassurance.

Moments in the Death of a Flesh Mechanic...a healer's rebirth

My hands and ears double-checked his blood pressure and found it stable. My left hand migrated to the little bit of his cheek that was exposed through the Velcro® strips, bandages and chinstrap that, cocoon like, wrapped his upper torso. My hand landed reassuringly where he could feel it. My mouth spoke, "Okay, John, you rest."

"We're about three minutes out," Jim called from the cab; "Is everything okay back there?"

"Yes," I said as my eyes moved over to Kathy.

I reached back to the drug box, closed it, and slid it between the gurney and squad bench. Sitting on it, I stretched my hand out to Kathy. I held her left hand in mine, keeping my connection with John.

Everything had been done that could be done. A tension welled up inside me; an insight, a knowingness, a rock-solid understanding.

It was awesome, terrifying and jubilant at the same time. I ached for these people to live. And as I ached for them, I found I was aching for myself.

I wanted these people to hold each other again; to fight, to love, to share, the whole gamut. It is what I wanted for myself. In experiencing my own powerlessness against the forces of fate, I met my patient's helplessness head on, and had to come face-to-face with first Kathy's and then John's surrender. In those moments, my own surrender was inevitable as well.

To lose either of them would be to lose a part of myself, perhaps the part of me that insists on believing I will live forever. To acknowledge that I, too, must die means that in a very real sense, a part of me would die along with them.

Touching them, I pictured my own longing for life flowing through them and connecting them to me. Together, we were standing at the feet of the same force that gave us life. Now, we were asking it for the grace to have it extended; all of us.

I suddenly felt foolish. It washed over me. For a second, I had thought maybe I'd have the power to intercede, that I could actually fight for their lives on their behalf because they were unable to do so for themselves, and by doing so, somehow lengthen my own. In the end, I had to admit to myself, all I do is manipulate matter and live under the illusion that by moving it around either by my actions or thoughts, I can assure the continuation of life. I cannot.

None of this is in my realm, I admitted to myself. For in the end, if death is losing, then they will lose, you will lose, and I will lose. We all must lose. If there are no winners, then losing has no meaning.

"This is not for me to understand!" I exclaimed aloud in my exhaustion; in a plea for release.

"We're there now," Jim called out.

As we backed the ambulance into the Emergency Room bay I maintained my connection with my patients. At my very, very best, I mused, I was no more than a tool of something that happened to work through me when I let it. I was not It. I wasn't supposed to understand It. All I could do was reflect a very, very small part of It. And in this moment, I was surrendered to It and beholden to It and at Its whims as clearly as were the people whom I was touching. I could feel a direct connection between me, my patients and this It: *The Great Mystery.*

My head was swimming, and my body ached. All I wanted to do was lie down. For the first time in my career, my adrenaline was not up to the task of carrying me any farther. The ambulance doors opened. Within two minutes, Kathy was in surgery and John was in a room specially set up to handle neurological trauma. My part was over.

It was 4:30 a.m. before I got back to bed. I remember my first dream very clearly. It was of a pigeon hitching a ride in the slipstream of two cars as they barreled down the freeway. It didn't matter where the cars were going. All that mattered was for that one brief moment that pigeon found exhilaration in their wake.

POSTSCRIPT

John although still paralyzed from the waist down, regained movement, control and strength of his upper torso. He is now able to walk with mechanical assistance.

Kathy, after two years of tortuous recovery, is now living a normal, healthy life.

Thank God.

Chapter Four
CRASH COURSE

When paramedic programs were first begun in the privately owned ambulance sector, some of the only people who were eligible for training had histories that would singe your eyebrows. They were an odd mixture of wannabe Cops, ex-cons, borderline (sometimes active!) criminals, thrill-seekers, ex-Viet Nam Vets with varying degrees of post traumatic stress disorder, and, generally, people who were unfit for normal 9 a.m. to 5 p.m. jobs.

Working conditions, hours, and pay in the private sector were dismal. Many workers were there because they had to work somewhere and nobody else would take them. A significant proportion of paid ambulance "hacks" (taken from slang for cab driver) simply didn't fit in to mainstream American society.

The pool of personnel from which the private programs had to draw was limited to whoever happened to be on hand. Driving an ambulance was something people stumbled into rather than sought out. Because the development of emergency medical services was so sudden and rapid, many of these hacks found themselves thrust into the forefront of a brand new profession.

In the late 1950s and early 1960s, especially on the Eastern Seaboard, with the exception of larger cities, specialized transportation of common folk in a medical or traumatic emergency to a central facility was a newly emerging concept. Doctors made house calls. Most health care was still being managed at home or in a doctor's office. When someone needed to get to a hospital, it was usually a family member who made it happen.

Around the same time, funeral homes were becoming more prevalent. They began to displace the practice of holding the wake of a deceased person at home. Eventually, some funeral homes adapted the back of one of their hearses to accommodate a stretcher of some sort and put an oxygen bottle and a tackle box with bandages on board. The converted hearse became available to the families of their past and potential customers as a "courtesy" transport service.

Local police departments had a "rotation list" where, when an accident or a call for medical assistance came in, one of the funeral homes on the list was called and then it would send a hearse to the incident. If it did well on the call, it built a new relationship. If it did poorly, it got first crack at the body. Eventually, the interior of the hearses evolved into designs more specific for patient transport to the hospital. For the most part, ambulances not only looked like hearses, but, in the minds of the public, were associated with their usual function, too.

With the exception of limited police, hospital, military or volunteer services, for smaller communities this was the extent of emergency medical care and transportation for the sick and injured.

Populations increased; house calls became a thing of the past. Responsibility for health care moved away from the home and family into the institution; the centrally located hospital. Funeral homes were increasingly unable to meet the demands of transporting the ill and injured. There were some hospitals who established ambulance services of their own. Volunteer organizations began to become more prevalent.

Naturally, entrepreneurs recognized there was money to be made. They approached each of a town's funeral homes and, for a nominal fee, bought out the homes' interest in providing emergency transportation. They would buy one of the hearses if they weren't in the position to provide a new fleet of custom-designed rigs on their own.

Then, with that fleet of vehicles and an area to cover, they'd invest a minimal amount in equipment, manpower and basic training, establish relations with police departments, politicos, doctors and hospitals, and begin responding to calls. They would charge the users for equipment used and for services on a per-mile basis; just like a taxicab!

It was from this point that, for most communities, standardized response and dispatch systems evolved. This would happen with other companies in the same county. Over time, through attrition, merit, politics, or subterfuge, one of those companies would wiggle its way to the top and eventually snag the contract to service the whole county.

The primary goal of the ambulance company executive at that time was to get warm bodies behind the wheels and in the back of their converted hearses so all shifts were covered. The agreement was to provide availability 24 hours a day, seven days a week. Coverage, not quality, was of primary importance.

The questions in a brief oral employment interview went something like: "Do you have a clean driver's license?" "Do you puke at the sight of blood?" and, "Will you work 24 hours a day, five days a week for $600 a month?" You can imagine the quality of the recruits!

These green medics had to learn by experience. As time went on, they availed themselves of courses sponsored by the American National Red Cross

(ANRC). The initial classes in emergency training ran just a few hours — from six (basic) to about 20 (advanced). Still, their attention was focused on getting to the scene of an emergency fast, staying there long enough to get the affected person or people into the back of the ambulance, and then scream off to a hospital. That was the emergency care of the day.

A big leap came in the late 1960s when Emergency Medical Technician (EMT) training was introduced. This was an 81 hour course; a tremendous improvement over what had been a largely unregulated field. By the early 1970s, many states recognized the need for standardization and made training mandatory for all ambulance personnel. The focus had once been on regulating the drivers of emergency vehicles, now those who had the responsibility for the lives of the patients in the back were beginning to come under scrutiny as well.

There were pioneers notable in the movement toward advanced services. California, for example, first offered a pilot program for paramedics in 1969. For the purpose of illustration, however, I will continue to speak about the Eastern Seaboard as I experienced it.

In 1972, a 25 year-old drifter could blow into a town in Florida and, destitute, need a quick, simple job. In an hour, he could be transporting dead bodies for a funeral home in return for "three hots and a cot"; a room in the back of the funeral home and three meals a day. He'd find himself doing an occasional emergency run. What fun! Within a few months, he would have to get Red Cross first aid training.

When the funeral home gave up its interest in emergency services, our drifter, having some experience under his belt, could be offered a paid position as an ambulance driver for the new private company. In 1973, he could find himself in EMT class. He had no choice; most states were making certification mandatory. It was the only way he could keep the one job he's ever had.

In 1974, a local doctor would decide to put a paramedic program into the hospital and hustle for funds and equipment to give it life. He'd ask the ambulance company owners, "Who's been running emergencies longest?" Next thing you know, our drifter could be eligible to become a paramedic.

People like these turned into, in many cases, reluctant trailblazers. They had no choice. Budding programs had to work with the people who had the most experience. For those with time invested the only option was to adapt or lose the job. For many of them, it was also their one shot at stability and respectability. The transition from corpse delivery boy to paid, professional paramedic — a period of about three years — seemed lightning fast at the time.

This new breed of medical support personnel had to be major hustlers or the program would fail. Literally thrust into positions of extremely high responsibility, many adapted well to the transition and became real role models for the new people entering the field. For just as many, however, the responsibility they had was not matched by their ability to carry it out.

They lived under constant scrutiny. The specialty came upon the scene so rapidly that even existing emergency support services were barely prepared to adjust to the change in the way of thinking. In the light of that watchful eye, many of the earliest medics crumbled under the pressure, or freaked out in one manner or another during off times.

As an example, for about nine months during 1977, I was the only remaining active paramedic on the shoreline coast of Florida from St. Petersburg to Cape Canaveral. Two of the paramedics who had graduated from the first class of the pilot program had been fired, one after having been jailed for impersonating a police officer. Another lapsed into drug addiction and was caught stealing a patient's medications. Still another burned out — literally "spooked" by the responsibility — and the last left shortly after having been given poor reviews for defibrillating a patient improperly; using no lubricant and placing the paddles in reversed position, leaving burn marks on his deceased patient's body.

Luckily, most of this happened quietly, and the public was not aware of these early growing pangs. In the hospital emergency rooms, however, the former drifters who did survive, of whom I was one, had to start from scratch building trust as if the program had never begun.

In the streets, an ambulance became more than just a meat wagon, and now, medics had to be more than hacks. Everyone was accustomed to the ambulance arriving on the scene, the "attendants" jumping out, loading the victims into the back and streaking away. Now, these young men — and in those days a woman medic was nonexistent — had to establish their territory and refuse to move until the patients were stable for transport. Medics had to spend time defending what they were doing and why. It included educating the people on the scene *while* the work was being done, otherwise, they'd be interfered with!

Medics had to prove themselves to each and every doctor with whom they worked in the emergency room. If a doctor worked in an ER it did not mean he believed in the program, or even trusted his medics. Unless they gained their confidence, and the confidence of every other individual in the allied protective agencies in their communities, they would literally be prevented from doing their work *at the scene*!

As a result, the medics who survived were smooth, streetwise schmoozers, but they also had to deliver. They were the ones who could do the work, and when they had to, talk their way into the hearts of citizens, politicians, cops, firemen and doctors and nurses and out of troublesome situations that would cripple the best of us. They had to know when it was essential to act and not back down. They had to learn how to get what they wanted, which was to be able to use everything they were taught to help save a life. But bravado alone would simply not work. When it came to knowing medical procedures, they had to have it together. The stakes were too high.

Many of the personal characteristics necessary to pull this all off looked like the height of arrogance. For many thrust into the profession, self-esteem issues were rampant, and most were driven to hold on to their hard-won and newly found status. But it was much more than fractured egos at work. Trained to work at an advanced level; functioning at a lesser capacity seemed absurd. The medics honestly fought for the right to do their best.

In a profession where financial rewards were nonexistent and the chance of receiving any kind of recognition was remote, the primary rewards were either in the quiet satisfaction of saving a life or the loud stroking of one's own ego. Did I mention that silence was not an attribute of the early medics? Here's a little story used to illustrate this:

A fireman died, like we all must, and found himself standing in a tremendously long line outside of the Pearly Gates. It took millennia to move even the slightest bit forward.

He was growing impatient. After much waiting, he noticed a guy dressed in uniform, stethoscope slung around his neck and carrying a cardiac monitor/defibrillator. The man arrogantly walked *alongside* the line and right up to Saint Peter. He said a couple of words to the Holy Gatekeeper, and without any delay, he was let in.

The fireman was flabbergasted. He said, "Hell, I went through paramedic training!" Pulling himself out of line, he boldly marched up to the gates and Saint Peter.

Saint Peter put out his strong hand to stop him. The fireman announced, "I saw you let that guy come through. Let me in; I'm a paramedic, too!"

Saint Peter laughed aloud and replied, "Don't be a ninny, you worm. That *was* God! He just *thinks* He's a paramedic!"

It's important to re-emphasize that as fractured as many of the personalities of the pioneers were, there were enough who adapted to and embraced the responsibilities of the profession to make it stick.

Once pioneering systems were in place and had been found to be viable, almost overnight ambulance services across the U.S. went from basic first aid to paramedic level of service. Transformation did take a good 10 years, fueled by the success of pilot programs here and there, but when they hit a community, it was like lightning striking!

The television program *Emergency!* which began airing in 1971, was a hugely successful show. It was incredibly effective in publicizing paramedic services. Seemingly from out of nowhere huge sums of money became available for new programs. Communities, volunteers, hospitals, fire departments and private firms across the nation clamored for a piece of the pie. Specialized equipment was added to ambulances at a cost of about $6,000 per unit and training programs were begun in rural and metropolitan areas.

What happened next was a shift that disturbed many of the original, seasoned medics. The character of selection criteria and training programs was altered significantly to fill this emerging need.

By 1980, people could graduate from high school, go right into EMT class with no more than a verbal okay from a sponsor service, and move directly into paramedic training. Within about 110 *days* a man or woman (and by the 1980s, women were breaking in) who had only spent a few mandatory hours as an observer in the back of an ambulance to fulfill EMT requirements could find him or herself providing advanced emergency medical care in the field!

As paramedic trainees, they'd start working supervised by a county-approved training officer. Additionally, certification would not be complete until they successfully finished about 500 hours of monitored field experience, which included a checklist of all pertinent procedures. Still, during that time, were there an incident involving multiple patients, the trainee would be on his or her own out of necessity. And making it through one new type of call, one time, doesn't mean you've got it down.

A typical work "shift" was twenty-four hours. You could work 24 on, 24 off; 48 on, 48 off; or 72 on, 72 off, depending on the system. Each hour of a shift (including sleep!) was counted in internship time requirements. Those 500 hours could theoretically be accomplished in as little as one and one-half months!

This was a grand departure for those who had invested years of their lives paying their dues on call after call where nothing but the basics were available; where all there was to use was your head, hands, and heart. They could not hide behind therapy, IV calculations, heart monitors and defibrillators. Endotracheal tubes and Ambu-bags were not an option. When you had to breathe for someone, you literally had to wrap your mouth around his and breathe for him. Most of all, you couldn't talk to a doctor and have him tell you what to do. *You* were your only resource.

Early medics had to hone their craft through tortuous trial, error and scrutiny. The new crop of paramedics began performing based on about six months of, essentially, schoolbook learning. This produced a really huge culture clash. The veterans, beginning from scratch and then thrust into professionalism, hid their insecurities behind cockiness, self-importance and arrogance. These same attitudes, however, were present in the ever-increasing crops of FNGs — "Fuckin' New Guys", taken from Vietnam veteran parlance. The only thing missing in the new crop was a twisted form of humility based on years of horrid experience.

There was nothing more disruptive than working with a partner for months, adjusting to each other and establishing a very effective working relationship and then suddenly finding yourself in the middle of a shift with a rookie. On one such day, I got stuck with a partner who was as green as they came.

Barry had been out of high school one year. As a nurse, he said, he could travel and get better pay, but it would take him two years to complete training. He opted to become a paramedic, something he could finish in about six months.

"Besides," he said to me as I started the ambulance, "I'd rather be through school and out and, delivering babies than do all that learning just to end up emptying bedpans in some ol' nursing home."

I slammed the ambulance into reverse and pulled out of the Saint Francis Hospital Emergency Room bay. It was two o'clock Sunday afternoon, and since we started the shift at eight that morning, he hadn't shut his mouth; nothing but dreams of glory and stupid questions. I tuned him out and let him ramble on while my memories pummeled me.

The call, some years ago, had come over the radio as a possible woman in labor, so I was even a little giddy at the prospect. Four years into my career, I still hadn't had the experience of delivering a baby. So much death and so little life! When I walked in to this house, tucked away in Shantytown near Daytona Beach, however, the scene killed any illusion of joyful anticipation.

Sitting on the top of a kitchen counter and screaming at the top of her lungs was a black woman in her 40s. She stubbornly refused to move from the counter and with her legs akimbo, I could see a *growing* bulge in her white panties with blood spreading out over it. She ignored my presence and bellowed to the walls "Not again, dammit!" Not knowing what else to do, I reached out and cut her panties off with my trauma scissors. A tiny baby popped out of her vagina into my other hand. That was the first and only delivery of my career.

It was a preemie that had been in the cooker no more than five months. It weighed in at about a pound and a half, most of which seemed to be from it being dripping wet from the woman's bodily fluids. I ended up doing slobbery mouth-to-mouth resuscitation on the tiny being, not having the equipment to intubate or even "bag" something so small. I used one finger to do chest compressions on it all the way to the hospital as I cradled it in my arm and up three stories on an elevator to the Neonatal Intensive Care Unit. That's where it died when the doctor on call said simply, "Too small," and pulled the plug. I was the plug, so I stopped doing what I was doing.

I was going through paramedic training at the time. and I was heartbroken. This was not the way it was supposed to be. The next day my instructor pulled me aside. She had gone over the case and found this was the woman's fourth late-term miscarriage in a row. "When a woman has multiple miscarriages, there's a strong chance she has syphilis," she said. "Let's get you tested."

Until the test results came back negative a few days later, and for years after, I gagged every time I thought about my one and most glorious delivery.

My FNG and I were on our way to the Polo Fields outside of the town of Carpinteria to stand by at a tournament. It was a lazy Sunday. I whipped the unit around a corner and up a one-lane street toward Alameda Padre Serra. It's a twisty-turny road that runs up and along Santa Barbara's Riviera, a set of beautiful, high-rent foothills from which you can overlook the city and the Pacific.

You can experience the great view, that is, if you're not busy worrying about opposing traffic on a treacherous road with no shoulder! Barry was tense. He stumbled over his words as he tried to brag how quickly he worked through nausea after starting his first IV in the hospital. I snickered as I thought back.

I started my very first IV on my partner, Riley, before I got into the paramedic program. He was a first-generation paramedic, having graduated from the first class offered in the Volusia County, Florida, pilot program. I was in the third class. We had a deal. I'd start one on him; then he'd start one on me. I went for the easiest, juiciest vein I could find on his forearm.

I fumbled. My needle went right through. Nonplussed, Riley had me take out the needle, and he stuck a two-by-two gauze pad with tape over it. Then, before I knew what happened, he grabbed my hand, picked what I thought was the stinkiest vein in my body and hit it perfectly. Once the blood oozed into the clear chamber at the base of the needle, he placed a 2 X 2 with tape on it over the needle, pressed down and removed the needle. Just like that!

Before I could adjust, he offered me the same arm I had just assaulted. While his skin turned blue and bulged out where I had bungled my first attempt, he guided my shaking hand to another vein half the size of the first and talked me through "the stick" successfully.

I couldn't enjoy my moment; Riley grabbed my other hand. He found the wispiest thread of a blue line and went for it with a small gauge needle. He went right through it. Within 10 seconds, the top of my hand was swollen blue-black to about the size of a ping-pong ball!

"Thanks for practice," he said after removing the needle. Then he got up and walked out of the room, leaving me to tend to my trauma.

Apparently my foot had gotten heavier as I recalled the loss of my innocence! Barry had fallen silent and now was gripping his door's arm rest. I eased up on the gas.

My regular partner that day was supposed to be Mitch, who was a training officer. He called in sick, along with, coincidentally, a few other medics. In a shortage of manpower, I was stuck working alone with *his* rookie. Technically, Barry was to work as my EMT. Right now, he was working very hard to look like he wasn't working hard to stay calm.

Under normal circumstances, Mitch would be supervising Barry who would be performing paramedic duties while I functioned as their assist at the EMT level. Mitch had three years field experience. I had him trumped in time. Still I preferred to be on the side as support while he went through his training routine.

I didn't want to be a County Training Officer (TO). I can't stand paperwork. Over the years, I also developed a training style that, let's say, was off the beaten path. I'd been told it wasn't consistent with county standards. Besides, I did have a resentment problem. I didn't like having to teach the basics to kids who only wanted to get out there and use all the flashy stuff that they'd seen on *Emergency!* Right now!

Off the twisting Riviera now and across straight back roads past the somnolent Montecito Country Club, Barry mercifully remained silent and buried his head in a textbook. We parked at the south end of the oval polo field. I pulled a couple of lawn chairs I had stashed in the back and set them up alongside the unit so we could watch the action from the shade of the unit.

The hard bodied rich atop their Rolls Royce-priced horses trampling up and down the course leaned over just in time to make precise whacks with their mallets. I was admiring how good their posture was, even when contorting to make their attack.

"An old guy," Barry started in again, "with noisy lungs, they say start a pediatric IV on him, right?"

"Yeah," I replied.

"But, that's 60 drops, and a regular IV is 15, right?"

"Yeah. Per c.c."

"So he's getting more fluid not less," he insisted, "'cause he's getting 60, not 15, right?"

I was distracted. A couple of women pulled up in a beautiful shiny, gray Bentley. They got out of it and sat on its wheel wells to watch the sport. .

"No. It's drops per c.c. we're talking about here. It depends on the rate," I answered.

The first thing that struck me was how tan and smooth their legs were. The shorter of the two blondes looked my way. She shifted her hips toward me and spread her legs. I couldn't help but look.

"So if you slow down the regular IV to, like, eight drops a minute," continued Barry, "aren't you putting in less fluid than if you slowed the pediatric down to 15 drops a minute?"

Culottes. I looked at them and then up to the woman's face. She smiled at me underneath her sunglasses through deep furrows of wrinkled tan. Turning to Barry, I took one of my hands and spit in it. He was stunned motionless. I took my other hand and spit about the same amount into it and held them both out where he could see.

"Lookit," I said impatiently, "There's a c.c. in my left hand and a c.c. in my right hand. Same amount, got it? One Cee Cee."

"Uh, huh." Barry looked at me as if I were nuts.

"Check it out," I continued; "a pediatric IV breaks that c.c. into 60 parts. Those parts come out as drops. A regular IV breaks up that c.c. into 15 drops. Same damn c.c., just different number of parts to get there. So when you give someone 30 drops pediatric, you're giving them one-half a c.c. With eight drops through the regular IV, they're getting just a little more than a half c.c."

I wiped my hands on my pants and grabbed his left hand with my right and right with my left. I motioned like I was going to spit in them. Barry flinched. "Now, look at your hands," I said, not spitting.

I shook his left hand briskly, smiling at his shocked expression. "Your left hand is pediatric — 60 drops per c.c. — Sixty. Your right is regular." I shook his right hand more slowly; "Fifteen drops per c.c.; fifteen. Next time you have to figure it out, spit in the hand that corresponds. You'll remember."

Barry kept to himself for the rest of the polo match. He quietly went into the back of the rig and started going through the drug box, taking things apart and putting them back together.

The nice thing about doing stand-by at rodeos, polo matches and other dangerous sports is you get to see the injuries happen. For most calls, you deal with the aftermath. You put together a picture of what may have happened in your mind, but you really don't know the minute details producing the injuries. Witnessing it happen, you get to see how the injuries occur.

I covered Daytona International Speedway races during the mid-1970s. Paramedic emergency crews were issued an empty "civilian" van, a fire extinguisher, a backboard and a tackle box of bandages. Back to the hack days! We would load the injured driver into the van and race to the track hospital in the infield. Anything other than opening an airway (we were forbidden to mess with the helmet) or stopping obvious bleeding was done by doctors in that 20-by-30-foot pillbox.

Pre-race one day, I was standing around with the crew of medics before the race started. 12 of us were stationed one pair to a van around the track. I said something like, "Well, at least we don't have to put up a front and say we're here for anything other than the blood and guts!"

To my surprise, to a medic, each of them reacted as if I were nuts, exclaiming things like; "Don't be ridiculous; it's about the race." To this day, I think they were all full of crap. Maybe one of my problems is I think everyone's as twisted as I am.

Like most stand-bys, nothing of note happened on the polo field except having to check out one of the riders for a sprain, but I got to see him fall off his horse and watch another horse stomp his ankle!

On our way back to our base, we were deflected to another call. It was a woman down. The phone dropped to the floor while she was calling 9-1-1. The line was traced, and the address given to us.

We got to the home quickly. Barry jumped out, opened the side door, grabbed the drug box and monitor and bounded on to the porch. I expected him to burst in to the house, but he stopped dead in his tracks at the front door. Putting down his gear, he carefully stood to the side of the door and knocked.

As I walked right past him and twisted the doorknob and walked into the house, I said, "You watch too much TV; this is Santa Barbara, Barry. You're a good guy. No one's gonna shoot you!" I cheerily yelled out "Medics!" as he fumbled with the equipment and then followed me in.

Something hit me. If I at all sensed danger, I knew I would do exactly what he just did. How arrogant to deny him the opportunity to follow his own gut! For a second, I got a twinge of guilt. Was I being too hard on the kid? A fleeting impression, it passed.

Popping my head into a room, I saw a woman laying flat on her back, arms splayed, unconscious in the center of a huge bed. Barry came in and started putting the equipment on the bed beside her. I looked her over carefully. Her breathing, labored, was coming out in choppy snores.

"Barry," I said, "she's got a pressing problem. Fix it. Then evaluate her. I'll be back in two minutes. Have a full report ready for the hospital. Have out what you need to use."

And then I walked out the door. I noticed Barry grab his stethoscope and pop it in his ears as I shut the door behind me. Walking out to the ambulance, I picked up the "Orange Box" radio and brought it into the house and set it up in the living room. I sat down on a couch and checked my watch.

I knew why I wasn't a training officer. I was heartless; I had to admit it. I wanted everybody to go through the agony I went through to learn the job. I didn't want to teach him. I resented it. Yet, for two years I rode on the coattails of my partners back in Florida. Would I have been a better medic if they had thrown me into the deep end of the pool? I may very well have quit!

After four minutes had elapsed — and I knew how much of an eternity an extra 120 seconds are to an FNG — I went back into the bedroom. Barry had been fast at work. A blood pressure cuff was wrapped around the woman's arm. The drug box was opened, and an IV bag was laid out on the bed along with a tourniquet, needles and blood specimen tubes; all lined up just perfectly. She was hooked up to the cardiac monitor. He was hunched over her, listening to her heart with the stethoscope. He stood up and faced me.

Though I had started to feel a bit chastened and open, the second I entered the room, a ball of flame ran up into my head. I got angry. I found myself barking out, "What's wrong with this picture?"

Barry looked at me in confusion and then said, "Well, her pressure's 98 over 64. Her pulse is 124. She's wet. Her rhythm is almost sinus tachycardia. I ran a strip..." He held a narrow printout of her cardiac rhythm out to me.

I ignored it. I repeated myself, with more menace. "What's wrong with this picture?!"

Barry was flustered. His face turned red. "Um, I think she might be diabetic. I set out the IV. I'm ready to draw blood..." He pointed to the tubes.

"Something serious is going on here, Barry." I reached out and took the stethoscope out of his ears. He was sweating now. "Just stand here and listen!" I said, softening my voice. "Listen."

Barry looked around the room and to the woman. He looked at me. Suddenly, he jerked straight up. Eyes wide, he looked back to the woman. Something clicked.

"OhmiGod!" he exclaimed, "Her airway's obstructed!"

The woman's tongue was flopping back into her throat and flapping as she breathed; making the very loud, tortuous snore I had heard when we first entered the room about eight minutes earlier. He missed it, he completely missed it, so lost was he in all his toys!

Barry dove into the respiratory box. I knew he was looking for a plastic airway to put into her mouth. It would anchor her tongue so that it wouldn't obstruct her air passage.

Silently, I reached out and grabbed his hand, pulled it out of the box, empty, and brought it over to the woman's face. I stuck his thumb in her mouth behind her lower teeth and closed his forefinger down below her chin. Gently clamping down, together we pulled her jaw out and forward. The tortured breathing stopped. Someday, that could be someone he loves, and he won't have an airway box nearby.

"Jesus Christ, I almost killed her!" Barry moaned.

I gave him no time to reflect. Before he knew it, he was calling in to the hospital, getting orders, setting up and starting the IV, drawing bloods, and administering 50 c.c. of Glucose. I hooked the woman up to a portable oxygen tank. We both transferred her on to the gurney. By the time she was in the rig, she was conscious and alert.

At the hospital, I had Barry do most of the paperwork. I hate paperwork, did I mention? I did an evaluation of him on that call, though, and in the process, was evaluating myself.

Whatever anger I had felt before had evaporated. I've learned that it doesn't matter how many times you fall, or how often; what matters most is you recover. He recovered. I wasn't quite sure if I had.

I thought for a moment maybe being a training officer could be fun. Barry did do very well. He handled everything like a pro — for an FNG that is. Though, still, I was a heartless prick. For him there was the oversight with the airway, and for me, I put that patient in danger by letting that go on so long, didn't I?

Oh, did I also mention that I knew that woman? I knew her real well. That call was the fourth time that year she was worked up by my crew. The last time I picked her up she had been lying in that same bed, in that same position, unconscious as a flower pot, snoring that same snore...for two days.

Barry didn't need to know that, though, did he? Why let anything tarnish such a powerful lesson!

Chapter Five
TOVARRUVIAS

The nameless boy just laid there — arms akimbo and a pump doing the breathing for him. The pride of our night's work had become a bookend.

My partner Hank and I stood at the foot of the Intensive Care Unit bed and stared. So many years as a paramedic told me not to take it on. But this had been such a clean save, I thought; so rare.

I was sure this kid could have had a future. Hadn't we given him that chance? We replaced the blood he lost from the knife wound with fluids. Then, we restarted his heart. He was dead, and then alive.

In the sterile white light of the room, it came to me that we had reached into the boy's worst nightmare and by some twisted magic, been able to pull him out of it. But he was supposed to have awakened. Instead, he was tossed into a reality far more harsh than anything any of us could ever have dreamed — the limbo of being alive within a dead body. Or was it being dead in a live body?

I was barely sure whose dream or nightmare this was. Sometimes as a medic, I'd have whoppers of my own. They'd start with real experiences grounded in a routine part of my day, and then suddenly, they'd morph until I was in some sort of surreal vortex.

Any emergency worker thrust into relentless challenges over extended periods of time is familiar with the twilight zone between sleep and wakefulness. When aroused from deep sleep by an emergency, disorientation occurs where it's hard to tell what is real and what is not. This has provided the springboard for many of my most harrowing moments; some real, some — literally! — dreamed up.

In the midst of peaceful sleep, a distant high-low-higher tone would sound — the signature paging tone for my unit. It would repeat, gathering momentum and strength and intensity like a light coming out of the fog until my consciousness was nothing but the tone. Conditioned to sit up, pull on a jumpsuit and thrust my feet into my boots, I'd be up and out to the rig; at times, feeling like forty tons dragging, other times like a feather floating.

Moments in the Death of a Flesh Mechanic...a healer's rebirth

The signature of my personal nightmares was a blissful, dreamy state, an adrenaline rush of a feeling of life itself awakening in me. My heartbeat would pick up its rhythm; thump—thump—thump-thump, thumpthumpthump, and then I'd be in the ambulance.

I'd be on the way to a call...or a nightmare. In that haze of unreality, especially during an exhausting day, I could not tell which. Before I would know it, it would happen and it would be finished and I'd feel myself back in bed and drifting once more into slumber. Sometimes that was really happening. Sometimes, it'd be a dream within a dream. The next morning, on my way home from my shift, I'd find myself wondering whether what I experienced was real or some mad fantasy.

When I awoke one morning, I believed I had come from here:

My head had hit the pillow after finishing a 3:00 a.m. call, and then I was jolted awake by our tone. Silently, I blinked the sleep away from my eyes and moved, noticing Hank and I both were moving like automatons. The next thing I remembered was being in a smoke-filled bar. It was crowded, and a Mariachi band was playing loudly. Smiling, loose faces popped out at me through thick, rose-colored smoke.

I was carrying an orange tackle box with our drugs, and a Lifepak 5™ cardiac monitor/defibrillator. Two policemen passed in front of me through the smoky shroud of light — smoky solid enough to touch — snaking their way through the crowd, searching it seemed.

Not sure why, I followed them. The faces of the people in the bar were unconcerned. It was as if no one official were there. Unusual, I thought. In bars like this, the presence of uniformed people prompted a change in density of the atmosphere; a palpable tension of fight or flight.

The face of one of the officers came up and shrugged. He said something I couldn't understand over the din of the music and chatter like business as usual and we weren't even there. He backtracked to the door. I swiveled to follow and took a step forward toward the bar, stools all filled with patrons. My foot plopped into something soft.

I looked down to see what appeared to be a green sack on the floor blocking my foot. Crouching down to my knees, I touched it. It had hair. I yelled out, "*Hank!*" I barely could hear my own voice; the band was still playing so gaily. The crowd, oblivious, carried on.

Sinking down in to the surreal mist to investigate further, I spied a pair of boots shuffling. I knew they were my partner's by the zipper laced into them. Grabbing hold of a flap of blue pants tucked into one, I tugged. When I did, I felt his foot sliding. I grabbed his ankle to steady him. As he bent down to me, I released my grip and did a quick tactile check of the floor. Sure enough, there was a thick film of blood on it. There is no spilled liquid that feels quite like it. It has body. It has life.

We now were looking at the body on the floor, evaluating what we had. The band paused, and Hank spoke to an officer who had stumbled upon us and had also slid in the blood, "Get the M.A.S.T. suit and set up the gurney outside," he barked. The band started playing again. The patrons carried on as before. This dream was so detailed!

A few things fell into place. The body was face up on the floor. Hank checked for breathing while I felt for a pulse. Nothing. The blood was slick under our feet, and the pool was growing. I half expected the pool of blood to grow so rapidly it would overcome and drown me.

Hank turned the body on its side to sweep out its mouth and clear the airway. I could see "it" was a he. I pulled a laryngoscope and endotracheal tube from the box. Hank must have (Was that an "Oh, Jesus!" I heard?) seen a bloody hole in the body's upper right back, midway between spine and shoulder. He called something out to me, but I couldn't hear. He grabbed my free hand and stuck it into the wound. How did I know he saw the wound? Did I really feel my hand *in* it?

I became fully alert. Locked into the moment, my spine took over and my body began working. I set up the M.A.S.T. trousers and IV materials. The air around me suddenly got lighter...cooler. I realized the music had stopped. Feeling a hand grasp my shoulder, I looked up to see a drunk on one of the barstools. "Hey, Buddy!" he called out.

I looked up at a face that I knew had nothing pertinent to offer to this moment. I went back to taking the M.A.S.T. out of its box. Again came the hand, and again the "Hey, Buddy!" This time I let my hands finish their work as I looked up and impatiently asked, "What?"

Swaying, red-nosed and slurring; "Got a match?" he asked.

I ripped his hand off my shoulder. Were this real, would that have happened? Maybe I was in a poorly written comedy!

Now, my movements were tightly choreographed with Hank's, in rhythm with the frenetic music starting up. M.A.S.T. suit laid out. ET tube in place. Flaps closed; inflate suit. Feel for chest rising with Hank's bagging. *Right on, Hank!* Suit inflated. Deep CPR from Hank. I expect to hear a rib crack. If this were a dream, I'd hear a hundred ribs crack!

Move toward head. Open box, take two 1,000 c.c. bags of Ringer's lactate with IV lines. Interpose compressions. Grab scissors, cut shirt wrist to shoulder, wrap tourniquet, slap inside bend of elbow; vein rises! Big 12-gauge needle; Chest rising high from Hank's bagging.

The music suddenly stopped. The lights went on. I hit the vein perfectly, hooked up the line, ran it full flow and taped it. In the glaring light, I saw my patient was a boy no older than 17. Chest compressions were resumed by Hank. As if someone had flushed, the patrons of the bar cleared out, and with

Moments in the Death of a Flesh Mechanic...a healer's rebirth

them, the smoke and the dream. The cartoon characters were replaced by uniformed police officers and firemen.

I repeated the IV process on the boy's other arm, this time with a smaller, 14-gauge needle. The click and whoosh of a gurney being lowered alongside me and now there were eight hands being slipped under the immobile body and lifting it onto the stretcher.

In the driver's seat of the ambulance now, I hit the emergency lights but held off on the siren and streaked away to the hospital only a few blocks away. I called in on the radio: "Set up for shock-trauma. ETA; one minute. Critical condition male, late teens, probable stab wound to lung, bleeding out, no time to call earlier, Medic 4 out."

Hank's voice came from the back, "We've got a rhythm!" and I swung the unit around and backed into the emergency room bay. After a flurry of activity in the emergency room, the next thing I knew I was back in my room, my head hit the pillow, and I was asleep.

That next sunrise was my first of three days off. I gathered paperwork from the night before as I changed shifts with the oncoming crew. I remembered back to the smoke-filled bar and asked myself, "Was that for real?" I checked my clipboard and saw, indeed, I did have a call at a bar the night before. But still, it all seemed so strange.

Hank and I went back to the ER to finish our report. We were apparently too tired or unwilling to have completed it the night before. Once there, we found out some details from a police officer who had been on the scene and was getting his reports done.

Our patient, as yet unidentified, had been standing outside the bar after having been dropped off by friends. Someone came up to him. They argued, the boy turned away and the assailant plunged a knife into his back and then ran. The boy staggered into the bar and collapsed. The bartender called 911 for the police and then went back to serving drinks.

Now, the boy was out of surgery. The team repaired a rip in his pulmonary artery, a major vessel carrying deoxygenated blood into the lungs for replenishment. He was alive, but unconscious. His surgeon was a doctor who once opposed the paramedic program, saying, "We can't let kids do out there what most doctors won't even do here!" He had swing in the hospital and the program's approval barely escaped his opposition.

He came up to me and Hank. I tensed, waiting for a hassle. To my surprise, he said, "Certainly pulled that one out of the shitter didn't you?" He walked away, smiling in what appeared to be approval.

Those words nagged at me in an unusual way. Maybe it was the look on the doctor's face. I wasn't sure. I knew I felt proud of my and Hank's work. Oddly enough, I felt even a little responsible for this kid who absolutely would have been dead was it not for us.

These were blasphemous feelings. This was taking the work personally, and that meant jeopardizing the clear-headedness needed to perform. But sometimes there would be an unavoidable emotional "punch" to a call and I'd get hooked into an emotional roller-coaster ride. Oddly enough it wasn't the horrors that threw me hardest; it was those moments when I really thought I had done good. Every damn time, too!

Usually, when partners get up after a night of running calls, they arise, transfer the ambulance to the next shift and, barely communicating, go home. That morning, Hank and I had a bounce in our step and talked about the call in terms that were very unusual for medics. Apparently, Hank had been sucked in as well. We agreed we wanted to welcome the kid back; and why not? Hadn't we raised him from the dead?

We checked the ER chart to see what bed he was assigned in the ICU. We just wanted to peek in at this point. In the ICU, we partially brushed aside the curtain at the foot of his bed. A name was written boldly across the chart in its slot in the bed. It read, "Tovarruvias?"

I became aware of the rhythmical whooshing of respiratory support. I asked the nurse why there was no full name. She said the name they had taken came from a tattoo. Legally, he was still "John Doe." They were hoping someone passing by might recognize the name.

Hank stepped in and flung the curtain open. He had a central venous IV mid-collarbone, the heart monitor was attached, and he was intubated and hooked to the respirator. His hands and feet were rotated inward. He was unconscious, and his eyes were partly open, but glazed; classic decerebrate posturing. His brain was fried from lack of oxygen.

I realized this really was no dream. My duty was done, and what I saw was the beginning of a nightmare for the boy and anyone coming to claim him. I was crestfallen. It was too real. I looked at Hank and speculated we had the exact same expression on our faces; surprise.

Brain injuries were God's way of saying, "You think you can cheat death, but you can't." Hank and I had worked with each other enough to know we knew where the buck stopped and it wasn't with us.

Three days off, and then we began another three-day shift. Hank and I talked about the logistics of the call, but there was a tinge of pulling for the kid, too. When passing by the ICU one or the other of us would pop our head in to check his status. No change. He just lay there.

Just before we started our next three days off, Hank popped into the ICU. He came right out and said with annoyance, "The little bastard even started fighting just as we were backing into the ER bay! I said to myself, 'We did it, we really did it!' I felt him come back. I think that's what's bugging me. I actually felt him come back."

Moments in the Death of a Flesh Mechanic...a healer's rebirth

"Yeah," I replied, "Just long enough to remind us we ain't God." My words were cynical, but my heart was heavy. Hank gave me permission to admit, yeah, I really wanted to shake this kid's hand and say, "Fella, make this second chance good. I want the best for you."

So, without mentioning it to each other, on the first day of our next cycle at work, Hank and I automatically started our shift by taking a walk to the ICU. We went to the boy's bed, but in his place was an old man, lungs dry and noisy with emphysema.

"I don't want to know," Hank said. Neither did I. But before either of us could turn and walk away, Sally, the nurse who had been filling us in on the patient's progress, or lack of progress over the last few days, came up to us.

"Boy, are we pissed off at him," she said.

"I bet you are," I replied. "I guess we are, too. We were sure he'd make it. Guess the little bum just decided to check out."

She laughed out loud! Hank and I were startled.

"Check out... that's a good one. That's why we're so pissed," she continued; "*He didn't even bother to check out*! He woke up yesterday morning; just snapped out of it! We extubated him. After about a half day of observation, we transferred him to a non-critical bed. We tried to get information from him, but he kept putting us off. The second he had the chance, he ripped out his IVs and beat it out of the hospital. Before security could get here, he was gone." We were stunned.

"Don't you know where to find him?" Hank asked.

"We tried to get information," Sally replied, "but he kept putting us off. Nope, he's gone. Nobody knows where. He's 'John Doe' to us."

"I bet the tricky little bastard's looking to get into some other medic's nightmare!" Hank mumbled the words and chuckled.

Sally looked at Hank quizzically. She didn't have a clue as to what he was talking about. I knew exactly what he meant. We were partners. It was our job to share nightmares.

Chapter Six
GETTING ACROSS

The paramedic system most simply can be explained by scrambling words. Prior to the 1970s, the operating philosophy of emergency care and transportation was very simple: *The more quickly you get the **victim** to the hospital, the better the chances are for recovery.*

After the introduction of pilot paramedic programs, however, conventional wisdom shifted. It then became: *The more quickly you get the **hospital** to the patient, the better the chances are for recovery.*

Note a not so subtle change in terminology. Prior to the advent of the Emergency Medical Technician level of pre-hospital care, the person for whom emergency care was being rendered was called a "victim." With EMT level of care, there was a concerted effort by the Red Cross (ANRC) and its instructors to change that way of speaking, therefore, thinking. It wasn't until the time paramedic services became prevalent that the switch to using "*patient*" was complete.

The major resource of the hospital is the physician. In some of the earliest pilot programs — Miami, Florida in the mid-1960s, as example — a doctor would ride in the ambulance with a nurse or medical technician and either render emergency care himself or direct the therapies given on the scene. There was a significant reduction in morbidity and mortality of the patients. Medical science had progressed to the point where afflictions once considered fatal were now treatable, provided proper therapy could be instituted in a timely fashion.

Certain disruptions in the electrical activity of the heart, as example, render it ineffective, leading to death. These are called "arrhythmias," meaning without rhythm. That doesn't mean the heart is not beating. It means the rhythm is not functional enough to supply blood to the vital organs as needed. In simplistic terms, the heart is beating too fast, too slow, skipping beats, quivering, or not beating at all.

Moments in the Death of a Flesh Mechanic...a healer's rebirth

These rhythms are identifiable by an oscilloscope that translates electrical impulses into the image of a "wave": a cardiac monitor. It produces a printed "rhythm strip" of the image up on the screen.

Monitoring through electrocardiograms makes disruptions easy to spot. Simple therapeutic action, such as the administration of certain drugs, or electrically "shocking" the heart using a defibrillator could reverse deadly processes almost instantaneously, thereby saving a life. Such things were being done in hospitals on a daily basis at the time.

Much of the equipment necessary to diagnose and reverse these electrical cardiac malfunctions, however, was cumbersome. Taking them out of the hospital wasn't an option. Taking the doctor out of the hospital didn't make sense either. But the rapid technological advances made through the US space program was about to change all that.

The paramedic program was the stepchild of improvements in micro-circuitry and communication technology that were a direct result of advances made during the push to reach the moon. Without this sudden surge in technology, it would have taken many more years for paramedic systems as we know them to have been developed.

Each ounce of weight in the space capsule had to have purpose. Miniaturization was essential. A big concern was how the heart would react to the stresses of lift-off, orbit, re-entry and touch-down. Cardiac monitoring equipment once weighing in at more than 100 pounds was made portable at a weight that could be useful in those tiny confines.

That was only part of the story. Another breakthrough was in placing two-way radio communication in to a portable, reliable package. These were radios that could communicate with a base station or each other without the need to lay down wires. These, too, were developed through the space program. But where they got practical application, and were tested under extreme field conditions, was the war in Vietnam.

Radio communication in war was not used for saving lives by extending the doctor's reach. Medics in the field made their own decisions within the limits of their training, experience and equipment. The value of the radio was in allowing men under attack to call in for air support, artillery fire and medical evacuations.

In the civilian sector, by the 1970s telemetry equipment was being made more readily available to emergency services. The APCOR™ (Advanced Portable Coronary Observation Radio — "Orange Box") by Motorola, weighed in at about 20 pounds. It handled the voice-to-voice communications between doctor and medic and was capable of sending a "three-lead electrocardiogram" over the airwaves to a monitor at the hospital. It did not, however, have a scope that the medic on the scene could also "read," nor did it have the capability of defibrillation. The Lifepak™ Cardiac monitor/defibrillator weighing in at about 40 pounds served those purposes.

Both pieces of equipment were powered by rechargeable batteries. They were cumbersome, yet manageable, and of course, there were various models offered by other manufacturers. These were just what I primarily used during my time in the profession. By the time I left the field, *together* they weighed in at about fourteen pounds!

Today, defibrillators are the size of a boxed apple pie. They diagnose the offending rhythm and discharge the proper jolt needed to "jump-start" the heart. The user needs no training, only to be able to follow simple A-B-C directions, and push buttons that light up!

Many lifesaving medical interventions became, literally "by the book". For each potentially fatal cardiac arrhythmia there was a drug or sequence of drugs that could help correct it. For trauma, there was a protocol for replenishing lost fluids and stabilizing systems. For many emergencies, following a relatively fixed treatment could considerably reduce morbidity or mortality. Blood pressure problems, overdoses, diabetic emergencies all had effective protocols routinely followed by doctors and nurses every day in hospitals across the nation.

With these innovations in communication a new idea was born. Why not train personnel how to use these tools to report to the doctor? Under the doctor's direction, treatments could be rendered on-site that would revive and/or stabilize the patient for the trip to the hospital.

The ambulance could now be designed to bring the hospital to the patient. A trained professional could then utilize portable diagnostic equipment, share the findings with a doctor, be told what to do, and act.

The fledgling paramedic program moved to fill the gap. Its goal was to train personnel to function as the "eyes, ears and hands" of the doctor so an advanced level of care would be available to the patient as soon as possible after the onset of acute illness or injury.

These personnel were to be *extensions* of, the doctor. The most intensive part of training was teaching the medic to describe accurately what was going on with the patient. The program was based upon being able to communicate a picture of the patient to the doctor so clearly, the doctor would immediately be able to diagnose and order therapy.

The medic had to be able to describe the signs, symptoms and changes of the patient. The monitoring equipment had to bear out those observations. Being able to start IVs, administer drugs, and "execute" other therapies only came after succinct and accurate communication was made by the medic to the doctor.

In the beginning of the program, therapy was ordered only in the most obvious cases. Unless everything came across clearly nothing more than basic orders were given. In a short period of time, however, therapies in the field became more complex. As programs became more sophisticated, the arsenal of drugs increased. The typical drug box paramedics carry today holds around 35 different therapeutic agents.

Even so, nothing more than the basics would be allowed unless the medic had gained the confidence of the doctor. Time remained of the essence. The doctor had to feel comfortable that every second was well spent by the medic. Only then would more extensive orders come.

In any hospital that undertakes a new paramedic program — and such hospitals spring up every day — paramedics are still treated very cautiously. This is part of the professional dues that must be paid. It even holds true with each paramedic new to an area or hospital. They must "prove" themselves to each emergency room doctor with whom they work. The complexities of the orders given are based upon the individual paramedic's ability to inspire the confidence of the guiding physician.

Ability is not taken for granted. Even in the case of systems that have "standing orders," where medics are empowered to render specific treatments in specific medical situations without speaking with the doctor, the second there is any flaw — when the doctor expects to see a patient with "X" and the paramedic brings someone in with "Y" — the medic may end up going back to square one: having to start calling in to the hospital once again for every little thing.

All medics go through adjustment periods where they find themselves under close scrutiny by doctors, emergency room staff, superiors, and at times, even their peers. It can happen many times in their careers where all of a sudden, they feel like a rookie again.

"O.K., rookie, you've got 30 seconds." Brandon, my training officer, shouted out at me as he put down the APCOR™ radio telephone.

"What're you talking about?" I asked.

"Bruiser's got the stopwatch out. She expects the IV done in... Now you've got 24 seconds."

"Great," I replied.

I noticed a twitch in my hand as I put the needle at a 45-degree angle to my patient's skin. I don't do that, I thought. But there I was, nervous as a damn rookie and doing that.

I was conscious of holding my breath. I carefully poked the 18 gauge needle through her skin into her vein. Removing the needle and leaving its Teflon® sheath in the vein, I quickly attached the IV tubing to its hub and began the flow of fluids. The dextrose and water solution ran in to her at full speed for a couple of seconds while I carefully taped the tubing in place. I then cut back the flow to 15 drops a minute.

A crackling came through on the radio, and then the borderline shrieking voice of the Bruiser, Doctor Helen Dellaver, came through.

"Is the line started yet?" she asked.

"Ten-four," said Brandon, smiling a smile I didn't need or want.

Another damn doctor to please! This one held my balls in her hands. I wasn't annoyed until Brandon started the countdown. I'd be jumping through this hoop and a bunch more hoops for the next few hundred hours of working until my internship was over.

"No one from out of state has successfully challenged Santa Barbara County Paramedic Certification before," was what the head of Emergency Medical Services for the county had told me.

"Has anybody tried?" I asked.

"Quite a few," she replied.

No sweat, I thought. As one of the first Florida State Certified Paramedics, I'd been working as a Mobile Intensive Care Unit Paramedic for three years. My training alone involved a year of schooling along with Advanced Cardiac Life Support (ACLS) certification. Beyond that, state certification involved repeat testing and an additional field internship of 500 hours. I knew I could qualify for Santa Barbara County Certification standing on my head. I was cocky.

I had even overcome the objection of being an ex-con by getting, with help, CA Senator Gary K. Hart to intercede for me with the DMV and County so I could cross-certify from Florida.

What I hadn't counted on was politics and the eagle eye of a woman doctor who was mourning the loss of her babies. They called her Bruiser because she fought like a junkyard dog for what she believed in. Unfortunately, I wasn't what she believed in at that particular moment!

Her babies were the medics that I and my new partners had been hired to replace. They were the first set of paramedics the City of Santa Maria had known. She put her own job on the line to bring them in and invested many hours of her personal time over the last year to train them to her standards. Then the county went with another ambulance provider who was able to underbid the company for whom her babies worked.

At 11:59 on December 31, 1978, they took their ambulance and went home. At 12:01 January 1, 1979, I was on duty in an ambulance owned by their competition, which, like me, was there as a result of an underbid (no acknowledgment of years served in my paycheck!) and completely new to the area. Helen was on duty, and she was pissed.

So there I was, starting the New Year at 4:00 a.m., in the front seat of an old Chevy Impala wedged in a drainage ditch by Highway 101 on the outskirts of Santa Maria. My job was to start IVs on two Hispanic women who were pinned in the car. I had to crawl into it through a broken side window and over

Moments in the Death of a Flesh Mechanic...a healer's rebirth

the passenger so I could kneel between the women on the front bench seat. They were both drunk and only a minute earlier started to complain of chest pains in tandem.

At the stroke of midnight, in Orange County, 230 miles south, they figured 1979 was a good year to leave their husbands. Grabbing a stack of cash, a sack of groceries, a couple suitcases of clothes and a sack of Cuervo Gold they threw them in to the car and headed north. By the time they slid off the shoulder and went airborne in Santa Maria, they were doing about 90 MPH. The car flew over an abutment and snuggled into a three-and-a-half-foot-deep drainage ditch beside the highway so precisely the doors of the car were wedged shut by its walls!

Now, as I tried to work with a flashlight precariously balanced on the dashboard so I could see what I was doing, the Orcutt Volunteer Fire Department was cutting into the roof of the car behind my head, over the back seat. The tool they were using was a huge can-opener-like thing. I could see the tip of the blade poking through the ceiling!

Brandon, my partner, had two years' less experience than I, was six years younger and twice my size. He was having fun ticking off the time as he got orders for the second IV from the Bruiser. He ruled by intimidation, and took pride in calling me "Rookie," which I thought only happened on TV. The only medic switching from the old company to the new, he thought he was the saving grace of "the intruders".

He made sure we knew he was the Bruiser's Best Buddy. Without him, he crowed, we wouldn't have a chance. He didn't have to prove himself. I, however, did, and it was all too clear he loved watching every squirming minute of it. As he handed me the set-up for the next IV, I could just hear the Bruiser squawking over the radio.

"Once the lines are in, send me a rhythm strip."

The reason I could barely hear was that the firemen outside were making a tremendous, metal-cutting racket and the women were moaning, groaning and crying out so loudly that I had all I could do to hear my own thoughts. Perhaps that was for the better, for all I was doing was bitching and moaning to myself about my circumstances.

Here's a paramedic corollary for you: The amount of danger a person is in is inversely proportional to the intensity of his/her screams.

I knew damn well that these women were projecting the pain they would be in when their husbands caught up with them. Everything else was fine. I had done my homework thoroughly. I wanted to convey that to the Bruiser, but Brandon had control of the radio. He was choosing to run the call like a life-and-death situation.

What I really wanted to say, in the way I had grown used to communicating with my doctors over the last few years was, "Everything checks out with these women, Doc. As soon as we get them out of the car, I'll give you an update. That'll be in about ten."

Instead, I had to take on a different persona. Under the scrutiny of this mad, wounded Doc, and an ego-ridden TO, everything had to be completely formal and done A—B—C—D just like the book says.

Each and every doctor was a challenge to be overcome. Once you had reached a mutuality of respect, however, you could pretty much get what you wanted in the way of orders. If either of you didn't have confidence in the other, you could pretty much expect to feel like everything was three times the effort.

That gap was often bridged by just being able to connect with the doctor on a human level. Perhaps that meant a little manipulation. For some, it could be making them believe they solved the mystery of the ages; for others, a matter of knowing their favorite football team...or nurse. But you had to find the magic key. It made the lives of you, the doc and the patient more tolerable.

Every time a hospital base station was established, or someone new took over the chairmanship of the emergency room, or you or another crew totally screwed up a call, it was go back to the end of the line and pay your dues. I felt as if I were living in an abusive family. Yesterday, I was dealing with Mom, getting praised for doing well, and today, Dad rolled in, hell-bent on making me feel like shit.

To this point, I had successfully passed all the clinical skills tests and examinations that the county required, but if I didn't pass my field internship — and I only had one shot at it, there were no re-tests for people challenging from out of state — I would *not* be a paramedic. But I AM a paramedic, dammit! I yelled at myself as I maneuvered into a better position to work up the women.

The only thing that was in my way was this training officer, this doctor and her staff. I had to be willing to play the game one more time; and again until I got through my internship. Then, I knew I could relax enough to put the old charm back into action and get what I needed.

Then again, maybe my attitude sucked.

While starting to work with the driver's arm to start an IV, I leaned back on the dashboard. I realized whatever I was doing, it wasn't about those women. Wrapped in my paranoia, I was completely out of synch with who they were and what they were going through.

I just went no further than the place where I had things figured out. I was with a couple of middle-aged Hispanic women on the run, yelling in Spanish and English, stuck in a ditch and scared shitless of what their husbands would do when they found out. Period.

At this same time, the roof of the vehicle was peeling back. Brandon handed in the monitor. I was in the process of blowing an IV on the driver, so it dropped to the car's floor. I slapped another tourniquet on the woman's other arm, and she started screaming and flailing about.

The Bruiser's voice pounded out of the radio, "What's the delay Medic Eight? Does he have a rhythm strip for me yet, Brandon?"

"Negative," replied my macho mentor, "He's kind of fumbling."

"You sure this guy was really a paramedic?" She said it low, but I could hear the words come out in between the firemen's grinding.

Another 295 and a half hours and I'll be through with this shit, I thought. Then I said, "The HELL with this 30-second crap!" out loud.

Unfortunately, it was at the precise lull in the racket during which the Bruiser could hear me through the speakerphone of the radio. I just knew it! And then I blew my second attempt at the IV.

Mercifully, the firemen started dipping their hands into everything, and before I knew it, my focus was on helping them lift the women out. Naturally, comments from the firemen passed over and through me. "Brandon never blows an IV, does he, Manny?"

"Nuh -UH!" was the reply from Manny.

As soon as the women were in the ambulance, Brandon headed for the hospital, 10 minutes away. I called in to give the Doc an update. I had done rhythm strips on each; they were fine. As precaution (to keep them occupied), I put oxygen masks on them at the lowest flow possible, ambient air vents wide open. They may as well not have had them on.

Rather than state what I knew was going on, a 15-second blast, I relayed my findings on the women. I included how they were found at the scene (wearing seatbelts, car intact) respirations, pulse, blood pressure, pupil reactivity, level of consciousness, heart rhythms, the details of the head-to-toe trauma examination done on each of them ("Head, negative for trauma. Meek, external exam negative for trauma, no complaints offered. Shoulder girdle, no pain on palpation." and so on, all the way down to their lower extremities and foot reflexes), followed by a concluding statement, "Patients are no longer complaining of chest pain. No evidence of cardiac involvement. Scope still shows normal sinus rhythm on both. Absence of traumatic injury. Alert, conscious, with stable vital signs. ETA to your facility, nine minutes."

Maybe she'd appreciate thoroughness, I thought. Like a very proficient mechanic, I had learned everything about their mechanics.

Dr. Dellaver's reply? "When you get in here, you're going to be the one to start that IV, only I'll be watching."

"Too late. Doc..." I said before I could stop myself. I had to find some way to turn this into a respectful statement; that's not what started to come out, "...uh, that is to say, um...this one was tough, but I already got the IV going." Maybe she'd appreciate my can-do attitude.

The doctor simply commented, "It better be perfect, Marian Base out," and the line went dead.

I started to chastise myself for being such a kiss-ass but then saw I only had eight minutes to get the IV going I said I had going!

Dr. Dellaver met us at the emergency bay door with an orderly and two nursees. We worked together to transfer the women to hospital gurneys, and then we wheeled them into the emergency room.

The doctor closed the curtains between me and the patients. I could see through the crack her going through an exact repeat of the thorough head-to-toe examination that I had just given them.

After she was finished, she came out to me while I was re-stocking the ambulance.

"I'm going to be breathing down your neck for a while, but I want you to know that it's not personal," she said.

My Inner Brooklyn yelled "*Right!*" but my mouth chose to go a different direction. "I understand, doctor," I replied. "The new kid on the block pays his dues. I know the game. Don't like it, but there it is." It slipped out. I was glad. The briefest part of a second of self-recrimination tipped into a "that feels much better!"

We were suddenly looking right into each others' eyes. Without acknowledging my statement, Dr. Dellaver simply crooked an eyebrow as if she had seen me for the first time, and this, without judgment.

"It took me two years to convince this hospital to cooperate with the County to sponsor paramedics," she said. "The administrators told me the first screw-up in this ER and they'd ditch the program...and me. I hand-picked the guys to work out of here and believe me, every minute they weren't running calls, they were in here with me."

I felt like I feel when I see my parents fawning over my nephew — Why the hell didn't that ever happen with me? Never really had Doctors take me under their wings like that.

While still maintaining eye contact, I noticed she was wearing blue jeans under her wrinkled and blood-splattered, white full-length smock and her sneakers had holes in them. I was able to take all of her in at once. I felt open enough to, for some reason.

"They got good on my time and effort," she sighed, "and now they're gone. So I have to start all over again because I won't let incompetent medics dump their messes in my ER. None of the other doctors here will let that happen either. So, yeah, it may feel like we're on a rampage for a while."

There it was...starting over. There we were, doing the very same thing. Funny, I thought, she didn't at all look like a Bruiser. She looked a little frail. Maybe

Moments in the Death of a Flesh Mechanic...a healer's rebirth

even a little bruised, like I was feeling. I hated when I could relate to someone I wanted to despise!

"I'm pissed off," she said, "because next year, after you guys are right where you need to be, the county'll put the contract out to bid again. God knows what the next group will be like. You follow?"

"Yeah...I really do." That's all I could think to reply.

She handed me the unit's blood pressure cuff that I had left on one of the patients.

"When you called in," she said, "and gave me the results of the head-to-toe examination on the women, you went over each area, and if nothing was wrong, you reported that it was negative for injury. That took time."

I started to tighten my sphincter in anticipation.

"I like that; it's worth every extra second." She smiled at me with surprising warmth. "It helps me know you are thorough. That's exactly how I train my boys. Thank you."

She turned and walked back to the ER. I congratulated myself on figuring out the magic formula. What was it? If all else fails, be honest? Experience does pay? A little kiss-ass applied rightly goes a long way? I wasn't sure. Maybe this wouldn't be such a tough internship, after all. Maybe I was on the right track.

Still, I blew every IV attempt I made on each of my next six patients; an unprecedented career record for me. Whatever the Bruiser didn't ride my ass about, Brandon was certain to pick up the slack.

364 days after that call, at midnight on December 31, my company's ambulances pulled out of the County and were replaced by another company's rigs and crews. We had gotten underbid and lost our slice of the pie.

Poor Dellaver got stuck with another bunch of rookies!

Chapter Seven

THE OTHER SIDE OF THE TRACKS

"There were maybe 15 in the bedroom," said my partner Dennis as he drove. "This old guy was lying in bed cursing, 'Chingadera' this, and 'Chingadera' that, and holding his chest. His face was like yellow chalk."

Cardiac Mexican, I thought. A canning factory loomed ahead of us and then quickly passed as we continued out of the Santa Maria city limits past a row of mobile homes and then into farmland.

Dennis was obviously waiting for a reply from me. Since he never seemed to want to listen, I felt no need to respond.

Yet, to my own surprise, I blurted out loudly, "Cardiac Beaner!"

I startled myself. Echoing my partner's attitude was in jest — camaraderie; no prejudice on my part. Not around this Redneck! Still, the words rolled off my tongue easily, and with a smile, too!

"Yeah," he went on, "Blacks turn gray. Whites turn to ash, and Mexicans get chalk yellow. Anyhow, I knew he needed to get in right away, so I got down to important business."

Dennis was a funny guy. In moments like this, on the way to an emergency, he was talkative to the point of being annoying. Yet, at scenes and most other times in between, he hardly would say a word. And the words he did use in his times of verbosity would shame a Ku Klux Klansman! He was racist, but you'd never get that feeling on the scene. He'd treat everyone fairly. He was quite an enigma.

Outside the ambulance; strawberry fields whizzed by. Rows and rows of migrant farm workers were stooping and picking, stooping and picking. A few looked up at us as we passed.

"So the first thing I made sure of..." he winked, "was that he had insurance." Dennis paused a second for emphasis. "Makes sense, right?"

Yes, always the money! There was a period of time while working for a private ambulance company in Florida in the 1970s that we were required to

Moments in the Death of a Flesh Mechanic...a healer's rebirth

collect at least half of the ambulance fees at the time of service. Yes, right there in the emergency room after the call was run; preferably cash, not by check, and credit cards...what were those? No matter how gruesome the circumstances or unsuccessful the end result, there we were; hands out — death and taxes on wheels!

The prices were incredibly cheap by today's standards; *only $72 to run a full cardiac arrest, with unlimited defibrillations!* That was beyond the standard per-mile charge for hospital transport, of course. At first, the company couldn't spring a new service on people and then ream their bank accounts as well. So the company made resuscitation cheap, but made us collect cash to avoid no pays, their biggest financial drain.

I didn't flinch at Dennis' logic. I scanned my memory to see if he had ever hit up whites for insurance before rendering care. He had.

"I looked around at the crowd," he continued, "and said to myself, 'Nobody's gonna understand what the hell I'm talking about.' This was Guadalupe. Nobody talks English in Guadalupe."

That's right, I thought. No one speaks English in Guadalupe. That's where we were headed. I wished we would hurry up and get there, get our work done and get out. I didn't like the place.

"I yelled out to no one in particular," Dennis kept rambling on as we passed a little red schoolhouse in the middle of one of the fields. "'Insurance, what about insurance?' Everybody stared at me like they were a bunch of fish. 'Insurance, insurance,' I said again, '...the card?'"

Dennis was talking about the Medi-Cal card; government health insurance, Medicare's little brother for California. It was a blue card with little stickers on it that recipients used in trade for medical services.

"'Card, the card,' I repeated; nothing but dumb looks." Then, his eyes perked up. "I remembered the Spanish. I yelled out 'Tar-hey-ta!'"

Ahead, the railroad tracks bisecting the little town approached.

"Sure as shit," he concluded, "every one of those damn Beaners — all 15 or more of 'em — pulled out their *Green Cards*! They started waving them like flags; jabbering at me in panic. They thought I was an immigration officer there to send them back to Mexico!"

"Jesus," I said aloud. I wondered if this guy was for real. Still, I had to laugh. It was a good story. Anyhow, I could certainly congratulate myself on not being prejudiced...not like that, anyhow.

That sure was Guadalupe, though. Tucked into an unobtrusive corner of the county about 20 minutes out of Santa Maria, once there was nothing, then there was railroad tracks, then there was Guadalupe. Today, there's still nothing, those tracks and Guadalupe. Its homes cluster between dusty streets surrounded by sprawling farms; a ramshackle island amidst a sea of green or brown depending on the growing season.

It once had quite a rep. In the early 70s, government corruption was apparent, especially with the police. The town had the distinction of being a place where comfort in any form could be purchased.

A few times each month, the ambulance would be called to pick up someone who had been beaten (at times by police), raped, overdosed, or unconscious drunk. At times, the medics themselves would come home bruised! You sped to Guadalupe, entered and did your business silently, and then left Code Three with lights and sirens blaring. Most every county has someplace like that, if not a town, a section of town.

I had heard things had changed considerably, but that hardly mattered. In my mind, it was still a Chicano migrant farm worker town, economically depressed, of little significance, and a place for whites to stay away from, period. What more did I need to know?

All I wanted to do was get it over with. For some reason, I wasn't half worried about the call. My attention was zeroed in on the town and my fear of it. As soon as we hit the railroad tracks, I cut the lights and siren. It's best not to attract attention to where you are in towns like Guadalupe. It's terrifying to be the only whites in a crowd.

That was the part I carried big time. When I was in jail, the ratio was 80% African American, 15% Puerto Rican, and 5% white. The whites who ended up at Riker's Island, where I spent about one-third of my sentence, were primarily heroin-addicted second-story men — common thieves and "scrotes", as we call them in this trade. I wouldn't have anything to do with them.

So I couldn't have anything to do with anybody. If I hung with the blacks, the white guys would put me down, and no black man would cover my back. The same was true with the Puerto Ricans. And every one of those "others" experienced a certain glee at the white boy having to walk softly, looking down and shuffling his feet! When you live in a racist society and the tables are turned, then you understand where all that rage comes from and you see the fear that lies under prejudice.

My first surprise was when we passed a section of Guadalupe I had not seen before. There stood some glorious pieces of Victorian architecture proud, tall and out of place amidst the clapboard houses near the corner of the block. It appeared to me the early settlers of the area must have had a vision for the town that didn't quite pan out.

"Lookit that," I exclaimed. "It almost looks classy."

Then we passed a graveyard.

"Ya ever read the inscriptions on those stones?" Dennis bleated

"Right," I said, "once a month I take a field trip to do that."

Moments in the Death of a Flesh Mechanic...a healer's rebirth

"Bonanno, DeGloria, Menotti..." Dennis said. "Wops; that's who founded this town. Dagos. Like you!"

I tried not to pay attention to him in part because I was looking for the house, in part because things were getting a little unsettling. I didn't like to have my notions challenged. The next thing I recall was kneeling down taking the vital signs of a jaundiced woman who, wrapped in blankets, was lying on a couch.

This is the way it happens. I would fade out of whatever scene I was in on the way to a call and go into an internal space; preparation; a place where I was emptying, or trying to empty, myself. And then, there I'd be, with the patient and focused. My body had taken position. I had passed four or five bodies in the room without interference to get to her.

My expectations were scrapped as soon as I saw the woman was breathing normally. This was not the difficulty breathing call we were sent to; the piece of the puzzle we had been given belonged somewhere else. Being a good medic is about learning first to figure what pieces of the puzzle you're working with. There are the pieces you're handed, and then there are the pieces you gather. They may not jibe.

The woman smiled feebly. The aged, not-American cast of her face told me she didn't speak English. Anyhow, nobody talks English in Guadalupe! First, I wanted to see what I saw without juggling words. She was passive, yet fully aware and peacefully accepting my touch, so I didn't feel the need to introduce myself and what I was doing quite yet.

Her pulse was slow and strong. I couldn't hear a blood pressure. I noted her arms and ankles were warm to the touch. Assuming Dennis was gathering information, I went on with my evaluation. No one was telling me anything, and that was fine; I was enjoying the absence of directions, guesses or suggestions being shouted out as I worked. Sometimes it felt as if I were on stage and all the audience were hecklers.

Once, in Daytona Beach, while working up a cardiac arrest, in the room behind me, this raspy voice called out, "What're ya doin'?"

Not wanting to alarm anyone, I calmly called over my shoulder, "Now, we're putting a tube into her esophagus to protect her airway."

A few seconds later, another "What're ya doin'?"

"We're breathing for her." I answered as sympathetically as I could. That's not an easy thing to tell someone about a loved one.

Five seconds later, "What're ya doin'?" came the itchy voice.

"Now..." I said and then dropped it. I was busy!

"What're ya doin'?" This time in a shriek.

"Look, "I called out loudly, "If you're gonna keep this up, I..."

I twisted around to let the jerk know I was serious, only to face an African Grey parrot in a huge cage. "What're ya doin'?" it asked.

As I did my assessment of the woman, I formed the words in High School Spanish that I would use to ask her questions. I learned to speak enough of the language to at least begin any medical call.

Finished with my initial exam, I took in a breath and started to speak. I steeled myself for a torrent of words of which I only could understand one in ten. Once the patient figured I spoke his language, he'd let it rip. In reality, I could understand far less than I could speak.

"Me llamo Russ. Estoy paramedico. Ambulancia." I began.

The woman smiled up at me.

"Tiene usted dolor?" I asked — do you have pain?

No reply. She smiled. I placed my hand gently on her belly and pushed, looking for signs of pain on her face. I asked again.

"Hay dolor aqui donde empujo?"

She looked at me with a stoic, benevolent smile, but I could see neither pain nor understanding register. Frustrated, I swiveled around and looked for my partner for help. Perhaps she was deaf.

What I saw was a room filled with Orientals, staring down at me with mixtures of wonderment, judgment, and helplessness on their faces.

"Good Spanish, Russ," Dennis mocked; "Wrong part of town!"

I looked at my patient again, and my face must have turned crimson. The woman's facial features rearranged themselves from Hispanic to Oriental! What I thought was jaundice in my paramedic surety was the woman's normal coloration. Embarrassed, I asked over my shoulder if anyone knew what was going on. Silence was the reply.

I knew the woman was sick and getting more weak and distant each minute. I couldn't get a blood pressure. That didn't mean she didn't have one, it meant I couldn't get one. I re-checked her other signs. Her pulse should have been weak, rapid and thready to compensate for the lack of pressure. Instead, it was very slow and steady. I took her arm out of the blanket and found it was a tad cooler to the touch, but still warm.

I was lost. Whatever preparation I had come in with was lost, too. What would I tell the doctor? How could I get orders? I had no idea what was going on. Every moment, it seemed to be getting worse. Each time I looked back, I saw more Orientals coming through the door. It was clear Guadalupe had a sizable Oriental population because they all seemed to be coming to watch the white boys at work!

Dennis hooked the woman up to our cardiac monitor, checked the rhythm and then went into the crowd to ask questions. There was nothing life-threatening going on with her heart, but that slow beat was confusing me. My gut told me she was getting shocky.

No one present spoke English. Once it was clear we were lost, the cacophony of Chinese, Japanese, or Filipino, how the hell should I know, started and increased in volume and urgency. It was unnerving.

Hispanic culture was strange to me, but I had reference points to hang on to. With Orientals, I was completely in the dark. In my career and life to that point, I had almost no experience with their culture. Turning to Dennis, I explained what was going on. He, too, was stumped, but he did notice the woman was wrapped in an electric blanket that was on full blast. He took it off her. She began to shiver.

How did I miss that? I asked myself. I realized I was missing a lot. So much for the results of my psychic preparation!

Dennis and I spent about five minutes — the most we could spare — playing charades. We made motions like we were hitting each other to ask if she had been hurt. We made faces and acted out vomiting and stomach aches. Our American ways seemed to have no impact, but we certainly entertained them; they stared in rapt attention.

Often, English-speaking immigrants when faced with people in authority act as if they don't understand a word; especially if they have something to lose, like getting deported. But after a few times of getting played around with, you can look into their eyes and tell they're faking it.

I noticed a man in his 60s who was walking around the outskirts of the room. He had that look; I thought he might be jerking us around. As each moment passed without knowing what was going on, I became tenser. Taking a gamble, I located the man again and stared into his eyes.

"Look out! Behind you!" I yelled at him, without making any bodily motions. He just stood there looking at me like I was an idiot, and then he turned away from me. I sensed he was insulted. Maybe HE was deaf. The only person full of shit there was me!

Now when I glanced around, the rest of the bystanders looked as if they were doing their best to be helpful — crowding around Dennis and jabbering away in their native tongue, pointing and giving him what must have been very vivid descriptions of the current problem and past history of the patient. Unfortunately, it all meant nothing to him either.

Meanwhile, the patient was going downhill. Her arms and legs were now getting colder. When you can't get a blood pressure and you suspect shock is setting in, you feel the patient's extremities and notice how cold they are and how close that coldness is to the heart. A few minutes later, you check again. If your first check shows coldness up to the forearm and two minutes later the cold flesh is deep and above the elbow, the shock is progressing.

The woman's breathing was becoming more shallow and rapid. She indicated increasing thirst by pointing to her very dry lips and then to her stomach. Now I was sure she was losing blood, but from where?

Under normal circumstances, where the patient is marginally conscious, I would have just stripped the woman down and done a head-to-toe visual and manual examination. But I was afraid of how the crowd would react. She was conscious enough that abrupt movement on my part could be disastrous. The question of whether or not she might be having a heart attack also came to my mind.

The time to load and go was approaching. We still had no real understanding of what was happening and, under the circumstances, maybe just throwing her onto the stretcher and getting her into the rig where we could work things out privately would be best.

Yet, I did not want to move the patient until I had a handle on what was going on. Dennis was circulating through the crowd. The accelerating sing-song rhythm of their talking was burning my ears.

A particularly raucous group of four people came up to me. In the midst of their loud jabbering among themselves, one of them, a little man, grabbed my hand and started shrieking at me in his native tongue and then tugged on me, as if trying to pull me away.

"Dammit!" I yelled. "Speak a language I can understand!"

The whole room fell silent. His eyes were downcast. Pulling his hand off mine, he started to turn away from me. My own attitude was alienating the only people who could help my patient.

"Dennis!" I called out. "Go with him, please. I'm losing it. I'm gonna get ready to transport."

Dennis went with the man to a bureau. I did a tactile check on the patient's limbs to find the cold was creeping closer to her heart.

Dennis now had three people around him, and I could tell in his silence, he had their confidence. He raised a bottle of pills aloft.

"Propranolol, Russ," he called to me.

"Oh, Shit," I mumbled.

Propranolol is a drug that slows down a heart that, because of a disruption of electrical impulses, goes into bursts of rapid activity. It slows the heartbeat and keeps it steady. There's a catch; the drug is so strong, when the body loses blood and screams out for the heart to beat faster, the heart, under propranolol's guidance, will just defiantly lope along — slowly and steadily, as if everything were peaches and cream.

Dennis popped out from one of the other corners of the room. In his hand he was holding a large diaper that was soaked in blood.

"She's a GI bleeder," he said. "There are three more just like this stashed under a bureau. They must have been embarrassed."

I cautiously lifted her hips to find another such diaper had been placed underneath her buttocks. It was wet and red at the center. Not a fast bleed, but steady. She was bleeding from her bowels.

The pieces of the puzzle were in place now. I called in to the hospital emergency room while Dennis started an IV line in what looked like the last vein in the woman's body able to accept a needle. I got orders for a drug that would counteract the propranolol and help her heart speed up. It was administered, and then she was stable for the trip in. She still had a long hard road ahead of her.

It would be wonderful to stretch poetic license and say that on our way out the door, our Oriental audience showed signs of appreciation. That's never the case. And I certainly deserved no praise. We quickly drew a map to get her family to the right hospital. I was fidgeting. All I wanted was to get out of there — to crawl into the back of the rig with my patient and leave that stupid town.

En route, I'd try to get my bearings; re-establish my rhythm. Something had gotten in my way, and I was still reeling from it.

Like encountering a pushy person in the drugstore, Guadalupe grabbed me by the sleeve and didn't let go until it told me all about itself...and me.

Chapter Eight
GATHERING FORCES

We were forty minutes away from the Neurological Center in San Luis Obispo County, flying balls-to-the-wall up Highway 101, Code Three.

"Everything okay back there?" Jim called out. He was driving.

I looked into the cab and made sure he saw me smiling.

"Peaches!" I said.

Then, I turned my attention back to my patient. She was strapped on to a rigid backboard and immobilized on the gurney. The head of the gurney was raised at about a 15 degree angle, so the backboard acted like the hypotenuse of a triangle. Unconscious, she was intubated and breathing very loudly and deeply. Wrapped around her head was a swath of bandages about two inches thick, solid red with blood. Underneath them was a bullet hole.

It was my fifth call for a gunshot wound to the head that year.

In my career in the back of an ambulance through 12 years in three states, I had handled about one each year. That year was a lot different. Not only had I handled five, but each and every one of the people involved lived long enough to make it to the hospital and went on living for days after.

By the time this call came down, I was damn good at "saving" them, yet I carried a huge nagging question; "Why?" Knowing there was no chance of survival, it was still my duty to do everything I could to keep them alive.

In that moment, however, I was congratulating myself. I had become proficient at handling such calls. When number four happened within a few miles of the hospital, the doctors there gave me permission to stabilize, skip their hospital altogether, and go right to the Neuro Center 60 miles away!

And here was number five and *Do Not Stop, Go Straight To Neuro* once again! It was all so routine to me now. The wound had been covered; the patient had been laid on the backboard, intubated, and an IV line opened. She was then placed in the ambulance with her head slightly elevated. The only thing left to manage, really, was her blood pressure, which was sky high.

Moments in the Death of a Flesh Mechanic...a healer's rebirth

Do you recall the still photograph of a Vietnamese officer as he calmly pulled the trigger of a gun pointed at the head of his prisoner of war during the Viet Nam conflict? It was an icon of the times. What most people haven't seen is the full incident, captured by a movie camera. The gun fired, the captive hit the ground and then, out of his head came a streaming pulsation of blood that spurted up and out over three feet from his body! Spurt, spurt, spurt. *That's* what happens when you get shot in the head; your blood pressure skyrockets!

The hole actually provides a release outlet that prevents the brain from being literally squeezed to death by the pressure. This is what happens when a blow to the head produces internal hemorrhage that is not relieved. In this case, you wrap the wound, but not too tightly. You replace fluids, but have to be careful not to overload the patient's system. You intubate to assure a patent airway. If the patient should go into cardiac arrest, you do nothing because of the severity of the damage. In the absence of that, all that's left to do is to cajole the doctor on duty to let you administer a potent anti-hypertensive drug, diazoxide. It's a last-ditch effort to minimize brain damage from increasing pressure and to reduce blood loss through the wound.

This drug must be pushed into the patient's vein rapidly to avoid tissue damage. It was used only in the rarest of occasions, and then, only if the medic built an airtight case for using it and the doctor felt supremely confident in the medic. This rare occasion was there was nothing to lose.

The anti-hypertensive would work as it usually does, rapidly; dropping the blood pressure until the body said "Stop!" With many high-powered drugs then and now, we know what they do, but we can't predict when they'll stop doing what they do. In this case, the anti-hypertensive could reverse that tension so effectively the patient's blood pressure would plunge her into death.

I had already gotten orders for and administered the drug ten minutes ago. The woman's blood pressure had gone down from about 280/200 to 200/150 and remained stable. Now, I had a moment to wonder at something that was bugging me.

Can you picture having time to wonder in the midst of an emergency?

It's not much different than learning how to drive. In the beginning, you are super-conscious of everything you do. As time goes on, your body adjusts and thinks less and less. Before long, you're taking in scads of information and handling complex decisions and movements without thought, leaving space for musing. Repeated exposure to calls with simple "A" then "B" then "C" procedures provides lots of "spaces in-between" to work with.

Where a lot of seasoned medics run in to trouble is they discover time opens up during calls and there's space to fill. Disturbing impressions, thoughts or connections sometimes come in, sometimes from way back When! Because everything has been competently accounted for on the technical end, the disturbance has room to continue as it is, or shape-shift into another form.

At some point, each medic has to learn how to sort through and either ignore as unimportant or make the time at some point to face the deeper spiritual, psychic, emotional and philosophical aspects of their experience. In the moments during a call such explorations are usually not appropriate. The medic can either push the thoughts and feelings back, for review at a later time, or bury them...that is *try* to bury them!

The dominant, allopathic culture tends to deny the presence of these experiences during the "delivery" of health care. It teaches by example, from peer to peer, many different forms of suppression. Years of this often results in the individual having a backlog of experiences that were translated into feelings that were buried alive. The most powerful of these will dig their way back out.

They can be triggered by an event, like a similar call, or even the expression on a patient's face. They can also come out of nowhere and with no rational connection to the immediate situation. They are experiential "hits" translated into emotional forms that are real and surface when they choose.

The irony is, rather than experience making you *less* susceptible to such moments; it often makes you more so! The more competent you become the more space in-between there is. The longer you're in the business, the more impressions back up, in some cases magnify, and then show up during lulls. The accumulation of unresolved moments is the fuel that powers burnout.

I was considering the two hundred plus square miles of Santa Barbara County during 1979 through 1985. With the exception of that one year, there were maybe three gunshot wounds to the head in any one year, and they were quite spread out; perhaps one in the north county, one in the south and one somewhere in between. During that particular year, however, in that section of the county, which was only about five square miles, there were five!

There were three medic stations covering the region, with a rotating cast of about 20 medics on duty from which the Great Lottery in the Sky could choose. To make things a bit more interesting, the last three of those calls occurred within about a two-square-mile area. More exasperating was that I could find almost no sensible connecting factors among them. Almost.

One incident was white-trash drug related, one was a hunting accident, another Hispanic gang related, the fourth a suicide, and this last one was spousal assault. Each one occurred within different neighborhoods, different socio-economic classes, without consistent sex or race factors, and had different inciting incidents. And most telling, things like this didn't ever happen in any of the neighborhoods where they happened!

Emergency professionals are trained to observe, search for, and note patterns. It helps them have an idea of what they're getting in to in the future. They are always seeking connections that can help predict the unpredictable. Some of those connections, of course, amount to superstition — but that doesn't necessarily make them wrong! Of course I sought to see if there was some

Moments in the Death of a Flesh Mechanic...a healer's rebirth

type of border or parameter that defined the area containing the incidents. They did occur during a narrow window of time of about one year. Beyond that, the only link I could see from one call to the next was I was there.

"Oh shit!" I chuckled to myself; that was one fearsome thought.

Next was to search for a *reverse* connection of myself to the tragedies; like they really couldn't have happened without me. That's when I said "Later!" to the human being. The Flesh Mechanic took charge and repeated an evaluation of my patient's status; head to toe. The space in-between, thankfully, was done.

Everything was stable with this patient. We still had another 10 minutes between us and the hospital. The only difference between me in those moments and the me who handled his first gunshot wound to the head that year was I didn't feel obligated to fill the space in-between with everything I'd ever learned as a medic. Technical worry can occupy a lot of moments and here there were none. I knew what was up and where it (most likely) was going.

Fuzzy thinking had room to occur once again. I was aware I was in a lull that I didn't want to fill with what came up before. I couldn't even remember what it was, but I felt a residual knot in my belly and knew I didn't want to go there. I thought of medics who, in the midst of such intense spaces would whip out a textbook and study! No judgment; that's just not what pulled me. Couldn't picture myself doing it and I smiled to myself.

While I took the woman's pulse I looked to her face and then remembered the expression on the face of her lover; the man who shot her. In each of the five cases I handled, including this one, I arrived at the scene early enough to have had contact with the assailants. There was another emotional tug, then, choosing head over heart, like a slide show, my mind jumped to the face of each perpetrator of each gunshot wound I had faced that year.

None carried the aura of a willful murderer; surprise was too genuine. Willful murderers I've run in to don't register surprise though everything else shows up on their faces clearly. Connections, always searching for connections!

Musing complete, we backed into the ER bay where we were met by the neurosurgeon, unhurried as well. We went over the details. The patient was brought to surgery. He'd see what he could do he said. As it happened, he could do nothing, and that nothing was enough to allow her body to live for another fifteen days!

As Jim and I were cleaning up our drug boxes and equipment, I was appreciating how far my partner had come along. His first shift in an ambulance had been with me. Shift rotations, which were often and unpredictable because the company liked it that way, prevented us from working with each other for most of the year. We had been working together steady, though, for a month now. He had even been my partner for two of these last three gunshot wounds.

We could talk about the freakier things we experienced without worrying about being judged. It wasn't that medics didn't or don't talk about the weird stuff. They do, but for the most part, it's in the context of shock value, disgust, braggadocio, sarcasm, anger or vulgarity, and always laced with humor. Jim got a kick out of looking a little deeper.

"You get the feeling that wasn't supposed to happen?" I asked.

"What do you mean?" Jim asked, while wiping the gurney.

"Maybe," I said, "the only reason it happened was 'cause it was in our area; like if they had an argument in Lompoc, he wouldn't have shot her."

"Oh, the gunshots to the head being right around here?" He asked. We had spoken of this before.

"Yeah, that's it." I replied. I looked in the ambulance. Its floor was full of blood. "I mean...is it the land, or what?" Jim considered it for a moment.

"When I first moved to California, from Virginia," Jim answered, "I could hardly sleep. I was living in the mountains around Bear Lake. Everything felt...electric, like there was an energy running through the place. It wasn't like anything I'd ever experienced."

"Uh-huh," I scrubbed the clotting blood off the floor with a damp washcloth.

"Maybe six months after I was there," he continued, "I was reading a book and it was talking about how the mountain ranges on the East Coast hit about four, five thousand feet at tops. They're old; real old. They've gone through their growth state. They're wise now. What the book said was the West Coast is still young; the stretching, growing, restless stage where everything is...like a teenager, yeah." Jim closed the drug box and went to the airway box.

"So..." I smiled at him and the thought, "Of course! We're on the Pacific Rim, here...all the volcanic activity and earthquakes and shit. It's geologically young here, I get it. So *we* could really feel a definite difference in the energy of the places because we've lived elsewhere. Once I got here, I kind of moved my life in a different direction. So why wouldn't that extend to there being these little 'hot spots' that'd affect certain people like me certain ways?"

"That's my thinking, yeah," Jim went on, "in the big picture, yeah. Though I don't think they're necessarily permanent, the hot spots, I mean...not like it is like in the difference between the coasts, no."

"How so?" I asked.

"Well," he said, "take these gunshots, for example. I bet you next year this won't continue like this where they all cluster in this one area....or maybe it will!" He corrected himself. "But it won't be permanent, not like the mountain thing. That's all about geological time. The stuff we're talking about is more transient. Like this place is spewing like a volcano, but soon it'll stop."

I could grasp the idea of a geographic area attracting a certain kind of energy. That energy got expressed in ways that could be seen through the actions of the people who gathered there. That's the place where stuff like that would be coming down. I stopped battling with the blood on the floor.

"Yeah, that's it," Jim said. "Like whatever's blowing through our coverage area will be hitting somewhere else soon."

"Wait a minute," I interrupted, "That sounds more like a virus."

"Wow...yeah," he said as he reached in to check the remaining pressure in our oxygen cylinder, stashed under the bench seat, "like a virus...I like that. Maybe with people it's a virus. That's wild! Like, this Arabs and the Jews thing? Maybe it'll pass."

"You think?" I interrupted. "Look at those areas, though. The people who've lived there have been doing that forever. Those have to be hot spots!"

"Yeah, maybe it's the virus that passes," he said evenly. "taking the hot spot with it. Or maybe the virus gets *activated* once it hits the hot spot. Who knows? Maybe one day we'll wake up and the Jews and Arabs are all peaceful."

"Maybe if they *all* moved things would change," I said.

I put my wash bucket down, and got into the jump seat, a swivel chair that sits just behind the patient's head. Jim stretched his legs out on the bench seat.

"Maybe it's some kind of combo." I began. "Like a kind of gathering of certain energies at a certain time make certain things happen. Maybe the virus *and* the hot spot needed each other. Listen to how I got here...to California."

"Is this as good as the jail stories?" he asked.

"I dunno," I replied, and barreled on "This was the last year I was a medic near Daytona Beach. And the woman I loved, of course, is through with Florida vacation and goes back to her Mom's in LA before college. Got me?"

"It's about a woman. It's always about a woman, isn't it?"

"Nope. So listen," I continued. "About a week after she left, a humongous dark cloud settled over all the county like a shroud. The air was muggy thick and lightning bolts were streaking *across* the clouds. Not down, but across, Swear! You could feel that ozone buzz, you know what I mean?"

"You sure *you* weren't buzzed?" He kidded.

"No rain," I ignored him, "None. I ran four calls in that shift."

"So, that's about average or a lot..."

"That ain't important," I interrupted, "Each call was at opposite ends of the county. I was criss-crossing the county."

"And, anywhere you went, there was that cloud."

"Right on." It felt great to have his attention. It wasn't often I could actually play around with such thoughts with my partner. "The first call," I continued, "was this 18-year-old kid, living in an apartment, threatening to kill herself. We showed up, and the kid was a mess."

Jim nodded.

"So, one thing leads to another, and I say, 'If we leave you here, you're gonna fuck yourself up, aren't you?' She says, 'Yeah.' So I told her, Listen, we can take you in for psychiatric observation for 72 hours. That'll give you time. You won't be able to hurt yourself. But it's gotta be at your request; otherwise, I'll need to call in the PD. Is that something you'd want?' Her eyes lit up, and she said, 'Yes, please!' So that's what we did, got her admitted into the psyche ward, at her request. We didn't have to take her kicking and screaming."

"That's rare?"

"That is *rare*!" I answered. "Next call; way south, maybe 40 miles and it's a redneck farmer's wife sitting on the porch with a loaded shotgun on her lap. It was a major violent family. She called us hoping we'd get there before her husband did. 'Get me somewhere's safe!' she told us."

"And you gave her an option?" Jim asked, keeping right up.

"Yes," I replied. "One after another, in different parts of the county, two more people, for different reasons, had me bring them in for observation and *then*, one more for good measure came in to the ER as we were leaving!"

"You had to be selling them on the idea," Jim joked.

"No," I answered seriously. "It was as if the forces of nature had come together in such a way as to make everyone in the county who was ready to crack, crack, but have it happen silently, and without violence. And it happened to me, too. I just had to know."

"Oh," Jim said, "Here we go…it was the woman!"

"Yeah," I said, "and that was the very day I decided. I had to know. So, within two weeks, I closed out my life in Florida, packed up my motorcycle and moved to L.A. to see what was up."

"Gotcha," He said, then, with caution "and what happened?"

"Oh," I said, a little on the sheepish side, "In three days, I knew it was quits. I ended up in Santa Barbara, but that's not the point."

"What's the point?" Jim asked quietly.

Moments in the Death of a Flesh Mechanic...a healer's rebirth

"By the time I got the bike out to the desert, Arizona and New Mexico, just after Texas, it was like...I knew. I knew for sure it wasn't about the girl. And another thing...you know what happened the day I left Florida for California?"

"Another force joined in?" Jim was really tracking me; Wow!

"Damn, Yes!" I exclaimed, "Nothing less than an *Earthquake* hit downtown Santa Barbara that very day! And I didn't even know that's where I was headed; I thought I was just going to LA!"

"So," Jim asked, "what does all that mean?"

"Now, I *know* that the whole trip, that whole day, everything, no part of it was about her. See? It was all about getting me here..."

"You mean *Here*, here?" Jim asked. "To this night and this woman..." Jim paused and started to get up, "this bookend?"

His words stopped me dead in my tracks.

"Well...yeah," I said hesitatingly, "Sure, right...here."

We both got out of the back of the ambulance. Jim removed the gurney and then our equipment boxes from the rig. While he removed the sheets from the gurney, I got into the unit and swung it around, putting its front tires up on a curb. Then I took the hose, and, leaning in to the side door, sprayed water on to the floor while Jim, sheets wrapped around his fist, scrubbed the dry, clotted blood out of our night's work.

Moments in the Death of a Flesh Mechanic...a healer's rebirth

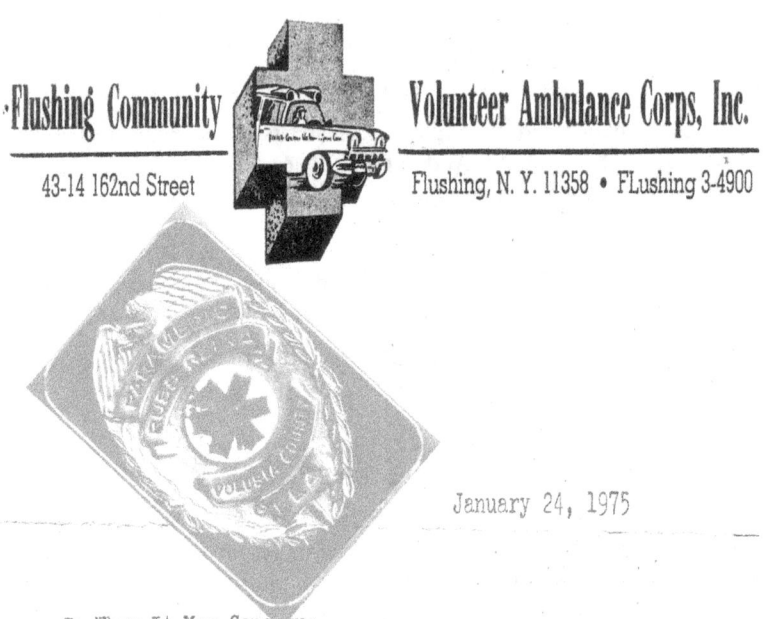

January 24, 1975

To Whom It May Concern:

This is to certify that Russell Reina has been a Probationary Member of the Flushing Community Volunteer Ambulance Corps since February, 1974.

Russ has taken courses in Standard First Aid, Advanced First Aid, Emergency Medical Technician as well as courses in the proper use of oxygen and transportation of the sick and injured. He has been riding our ambulance as a trainee since September. As of January 15, 1975 he was taken off training.

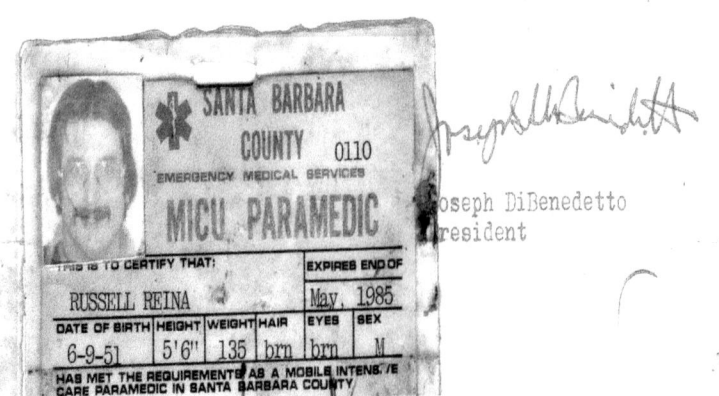

Joseph DiBenedetto
President

Moments in the Death of a Flesh Mechanic...a healer's rebirth

southeast Volusia by

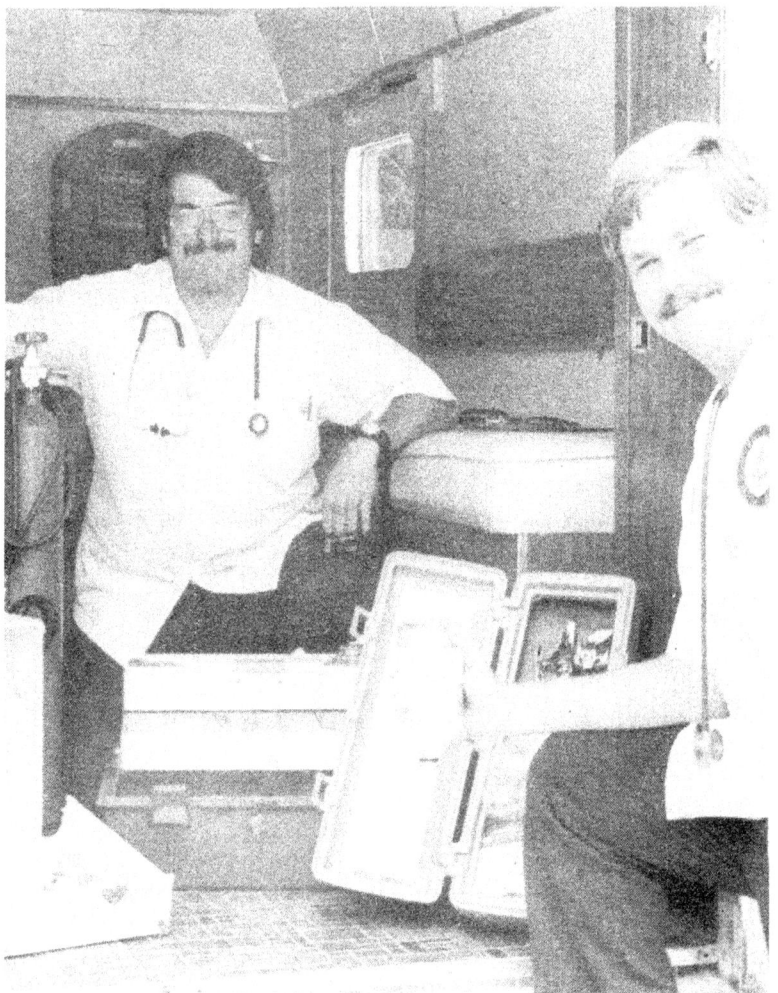

READY FOR EMERGENCY — First certified paramedics on local duty with Beacon Ambulance Service, Russ Reina and John Salmon display lifesaving equipment.

The shit-eating grins were because we were praying the reporter didn't notice neither our "Orange Box" radio nor our 40 lb. monitor/defibrillator had come in yet!

Russ Reina

BEACON AMBULANCE

> Notice: At the bottom,
> Beacon "Livery" Service,
> originally corpse haulers.
> (underlining mine)

1 - 904 - 255 - 2406
P. O. Box 6005
Daytona Beach, Fla. 320

August 18, 1976

TO ALL BEACON AMBULANCE TECHNICIANS:

    As you all know, we are preparing to engage in a trial program in which EMT II's will administer drugs, IV's and selected cardiac procedures on certain calls. We have recently purchased one additional defibrillator and radio to equip another telemetry unit at a cost of approximately $6,000.00. We have also trained 9 EMT II's at a company expense of approximately $450.00 per man or a total of $3,600.00. Thus far there has been no income to justify these expenditures which are well up into five figures.

    <u>I have no doubts that this program will save many lives, but as a business we must also look at financial facts.</u> We all know that the price of everything is up --- for example, our premium on Workman's Compensation Insurance alone was increased by $10,000.00 this year. Gasoline, tires and vehicle repair costs have also skyrocketed. <u>In addition to this, our total number of calls are down considerably and are far below our predictions.</u> This has reduced the income of the ambulance service to a level that gives us much concern.

    With this in mind I regret that it is not economically practical for Beacon to send any employees through this Fall EMT II Course. <u>We unfortunately cannot dip into equipment, salary and vacation budgets to train more technicians in a pilot program until we receive additional income either from the County or by an approved rate charge for these services, equipment and drugs.</u> It is hoped that this may happen in time for the next EMT II Class so that we can continue advance training at that time.

George Van Arnam
General Manager

Beacon Livery Service Inc. of Volusia Co...

Give 'em credit; the Co. *was* only charging $72.00 for a <u>Full Arrest!</u> (Much respect for Mr. Van Arnam!)

Moments in the Death of a Flesh Mechanic...a healer's rebirth

2—Santa Maria, Calif., Times, Saturday, January 5, 1980

Paramedics frustra[ted]
by contract termin[ation]

Out of work on New Year's

By Paul Engstrom
Times Staff Writer

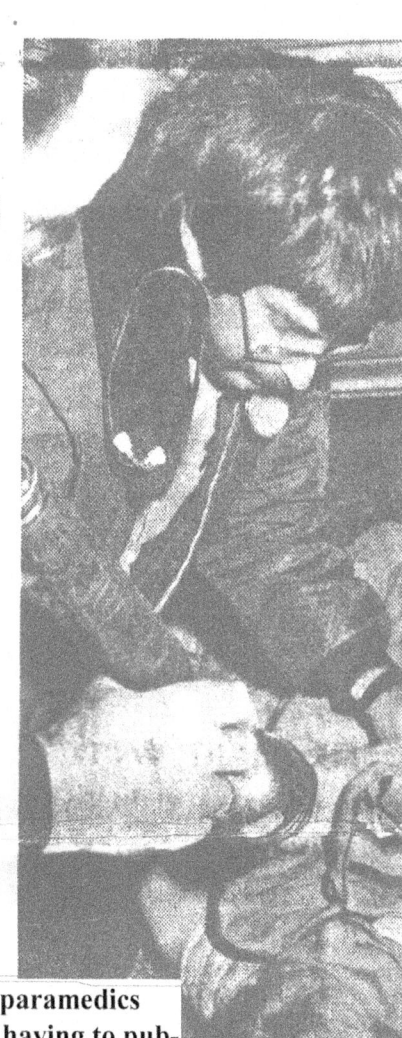

"I felt futility, just total frustration," said paramedic Russ Reina of the county's Dec. 28 decision to terminate its contract with his employer, the Mobile Life Support ambulance firm of Solvang. "I also felt remorse and self-pity. There was always a little bit of hope (for a contract agreement), but that hope was severed."

In spite of the gloomy news, Dec. 28 was a day like all others for Reina and the other 15 North County paramedics and emergency medical technicians. They could rave about the demise of MLS and joke cynically about their contribution to unemployment statistics, but the need for their on-call medical expertise would be a burden right up to the stroke of midnight Dec. 31, the day the ambulance contract was to lapse.

Ten years into the program, paramedics were put into the position of having to publicize their value and lobby for stability.

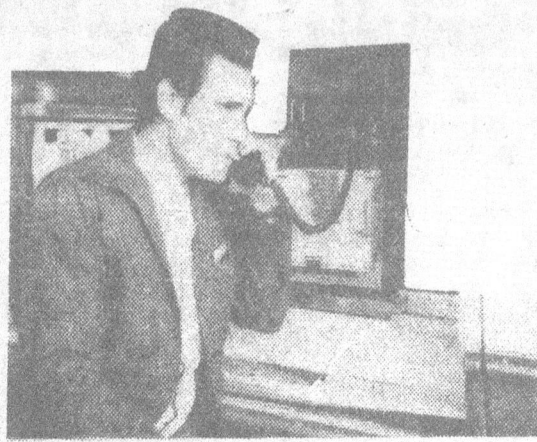

PARAMEDIC PROFILE

AGE: 28
MARITAL STATUS: MARRIED
FAMILY: 1 CHILD
JOB TITLE: MOBILE INTENSIVE CARE PARAMEDIC
DUTIES: ADMINISTER <u>ADVANCED</u> PRE-HOSPITAL CARE TO THE SICK & INJURED.
EXPERIENCE: <u>8 YRS.</u> PRE-HOSPITAL CARE.
PAY: $3.62/HR. 60 HR. WEEK
RETIREMENT BENEFITS: <u>NONE</u>
ADVANCEMENT OPPORTUNITY: <u>NONE</u>
JOB SECURITY: <u>NONE</u>
CURRENT EXPECTATIONS: LOWER PAY, MORE HOURS, LOSS OF JOB.

. . . THE PROGRESS OF PROFESSIONAL AND RELIABLE PARAMEDIC SERVICE IS POTENTIALLY IN JEOPARDY IN SANTA BARBARA COUNTY. WHY IS IT, A JOB THAT DEALS WITH LIFE-THREATENING SITUATIONS IS HELD IN SUCH LOW PRIORITY?? <u>ASK YOUR COUNTY SUPERVISORS.</u>

Paid for by: Santa Barbara County Paramedic-E.M.T. Assoc., a non-aligned, non-profit organization.

1980 ad seeking support of Citizens to prevent services from going to lowest bidder.

*

Ad by Mike Messina

*

(We weren't exactly adored by the county either!)

Moments in the Death of a Flesh Mechanic...a healer's rebirth

The California Paramedics Association was a professional organization. It contracted with the union to represent it only in bargaining with employers. We were autonomous otherwise. Unions were losing ground and compromising to attract new members at the time victory at the foundation.

1247 West 7th St. Phone 680-9567 2 Vol. 6, No. 6 June, 1983

Santa Barbara Paramedics send emergency call to Local 399

The failure of management to honor verbal commitments and a desire to improve the quality of their services led the Santa Barbara Paramedics & EMT Association to vote unanimously to affiliate with Local 399.

Secretary-Treasurer Gloria Marigny noted that although management of the 911 Ambulance Service recognized their employees as a bargaining unit, they refused to set negotiated matters into a written contract.

"This marriage of the union and the association will lend the weight of federal law and professional negotiators to the paramedics' desire to obtain their first written union contract, Marigny stated.

Union organizer David Rodich handled the precise negotiations between the union and the association which gives the paramedics full union membership.

The affiliation was finalized at two meetings of association members in early June. The lively sessions revealed the serious nature of the paramedics concern for providing high quality pre-hospital care to Santa Barbara residents.

An overriding issue in determining their need for union representation was the Association's belief that in a union contract, issues affecting their ability to deliver quality care can be firmly negotiated.

The current verbal contract between the Association and 911 expires in the fall which necessitated timely action on the part of the paramedics. The union and association members will begin to schedule meetings for the purpose of selecting a bargaining committee and soliciting contract proposals.

According to Rodich, the new union members are quite excited about the up-coming negotiations.

"The enthusiasm of these workers ensures the union of an active and informed bargaining unit throughout negotiations and the term of the contract."

The affiliation agreement was announced to the Santa Barbara news media at a press conference following the final vote of approval. The news was swept through the area as media representatives grasped the significance of Santa Barbara's only paramedics actions. The association had successfully kept the news from 911 management until they read, heard, or watched an account of the affiliation from local media sources.

Secretary-Treasurer Marigny welcomed the new members stating, "We look forward to a strong and fruitful relationship with these workers and will endeavor to assist them reach their goals."

Association members who played a key role in the affiliation were Dan Goldstein, Geoff Houze, Russ Reimer, and several other outstanding members.

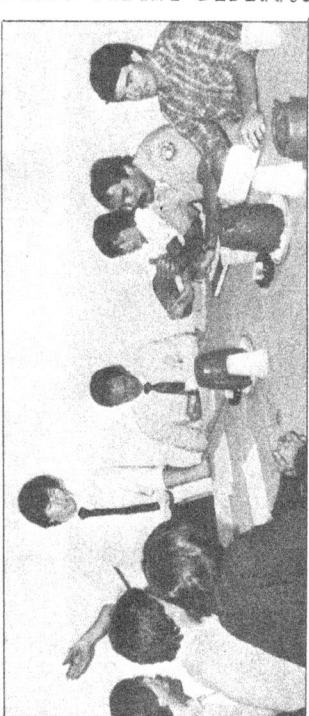

Santa Barbara Paramedics gathered to tally what resulted in a unanimous vote for affiliation with Local 399. Association President Dan Goldstein told the association board members that their action will serve the best interest of the workers now, and in the future.

employees from the Social Security mandating inclusion of all non- Although the union and its

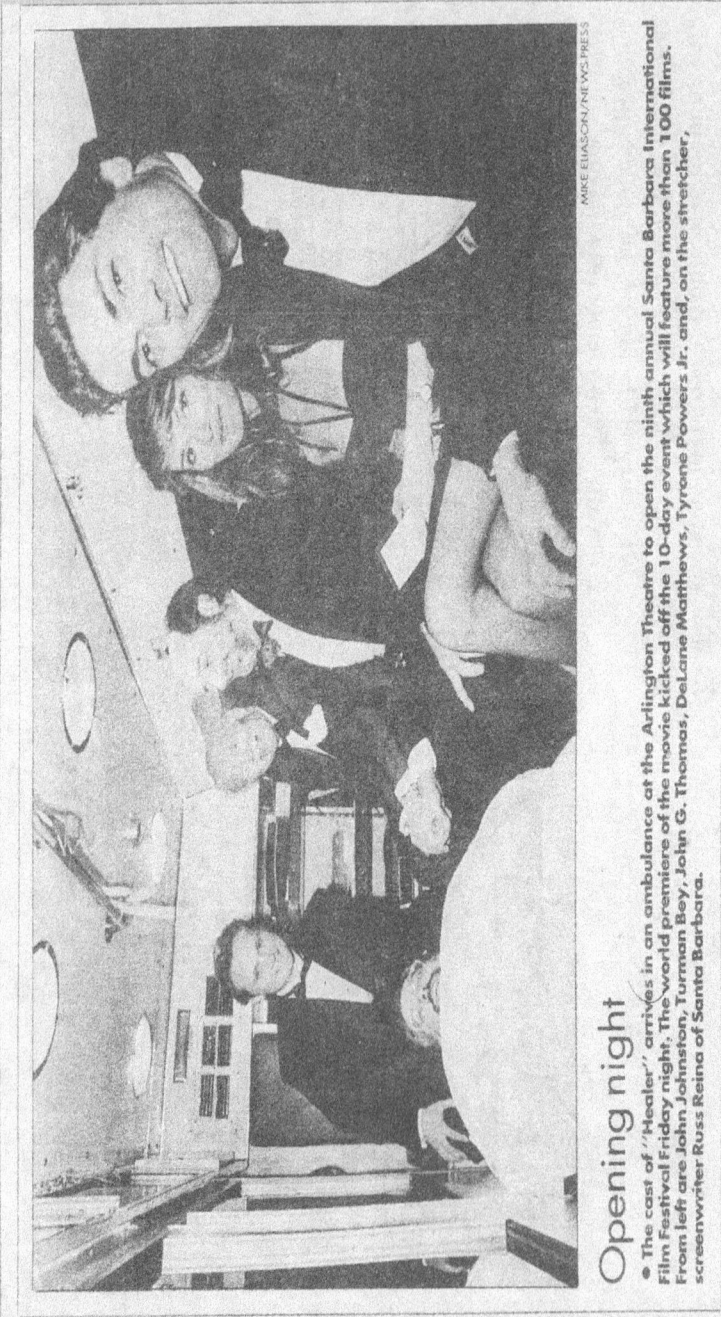

Opening night

● The cast of "Healer" arrives in an ambulance at the Arlington Theatre to open the ninth annual Santa Barbara International Film Festival Friday night. The world premiere of the movie kicked off the 10-day event which will feature more than 100 films. From left are John Johnston, Turman Bey, John G. Thomas, DeLane Matthews, Tyrone Powers Jr. and, on the stretcher, screenwriter Russ Reina of Santa Barbara.

David McCallum in *Healer* (1994), the story of a reluctant medic assaulted by the profession and people like David's character, the Jackal, an EMS abuser. It was a comic role and McCallum really wanted to "break type" at the time giving the tiny flick a stand-out performance!

The movie was a miracle; shot on a $350,000 budget! It was chosen to open the 1994 Santa Barbara International Film Festival because the Northridge earthquake wiped out the post production studio of a Hollywood Blockbuster scheduled to open it. Our movie showed, but was not ready. It's ready now, maybe this book will generate some interest and I'll get paid!

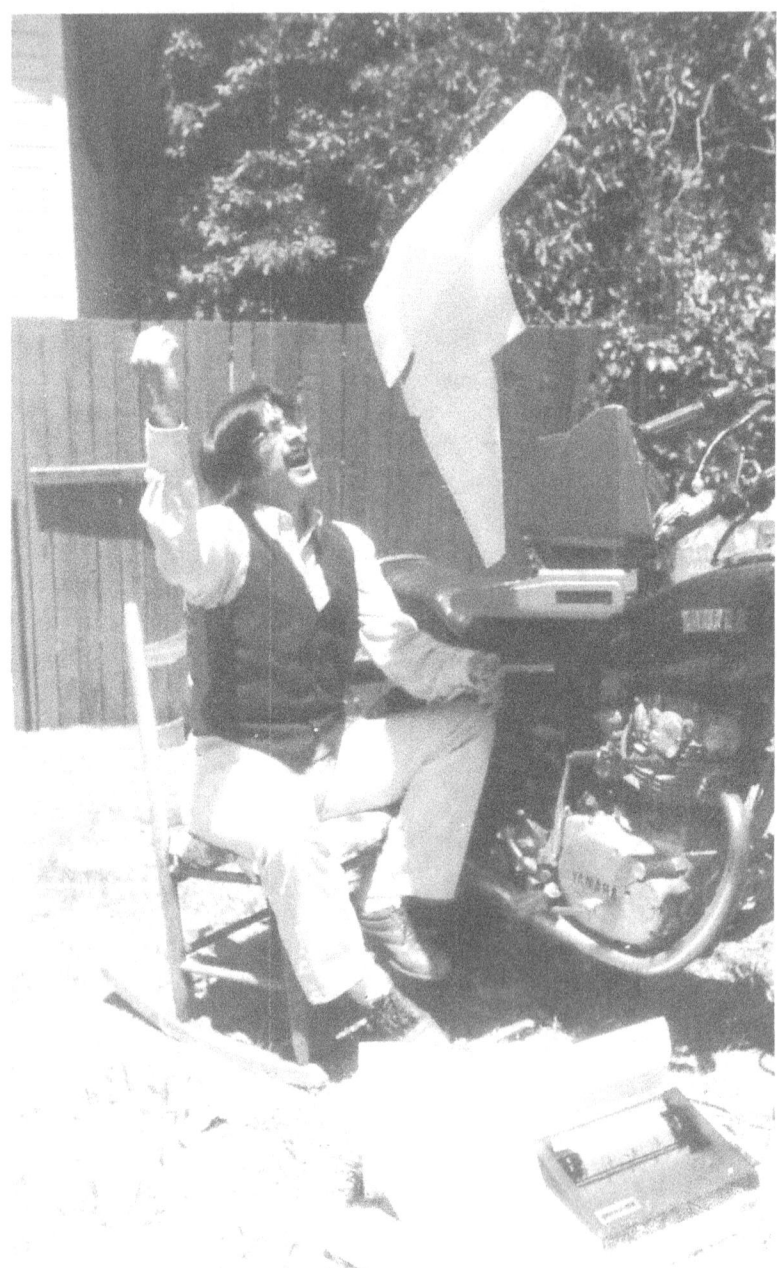

Someone just told the poor bastard that he'd make sense of the experience and even turn it into something useful for others, but it would take 25 years before *You* would get to see it!
(Note: The Radio Shack TRS 80 computer & dot matrix printer!)

Moments in the Death of a Flesh Mechanic...a healer's rebirth

Just so you know, I rehabilitated myself. Even though I am a felon I petitioned the very Justice of the Supreme Court (NY) who sentenced me to have my rights reinstated. I had to prove I was a law abiding, model citizen who had seen the error of his ways. He bought it! and issued me this certificate which reinstates ALL of my rights EXCEPT the right to HOLD PUBLIC OFFICE, which basically means you're safe!
(I always wanted to use this for something, Thanks!)

STATE OF NEW YORK
CERTIFICATE OF RELIEF FROM DISABILITIES

FOR COURT OR BOARD OF PAROLE
Docket, File, or other Identifying No.
Ind. 4792,4793-72 Cons.

This certificate is issued to the holder to grant relief from all or certain enumerated disabilities, forfeitures, or bars to his employment automatically imposed by law by reason of his conviction of the crime or of the offense specified herein. This certificate shall NOT be deemed nor construed to be a pardon.
SEE REVERSE SIDE FOR EXPLANATION OF THE LAW GOVERNING THIS CERTIFICATE
The Original Certificate is to be presented to the person to whom awarded. One copy is to be retained by the issuing agency, and one copy is to be filed with the N.Y.S. Div. of Criminal Justice Services, Executive Park, Stuyvesant Plaza, Albany N.Y. 12202

1. For use by DCJS	HOLDER OF CERTIFICATE			3. NYSID Number
	2. Last Name	First Name	Middle Initial	
	REINA	RUSSELL	J.	3514733N

4. Crime or offense for which convicted	5. Date of arrest	6. Date of sentence
Att. Cr. Selling Dangerous Drug 4°	12/9/72	5/21/73

7. Court of disposition	8. Certificate Issued by:
SUPREME COURT, QUEENS COUNTY CRIMINAL TERM	[X] COURT INDICATED IN NO. 7 [ ] STATE BOARD OF PAROLE

9. Date this certificate issued	10. If this Certificate replaces Certificate of Relief From Disabilities previously issued, give date of previous Certificate.
June 6, 1974	Date: [X] Not Applicable

11. CHECK ONE BOX ONLY
This certificate shall:

[ ] a. Relieve the holder of all forfeitures, and of all disabilities and bars to employment, excluding the right to retain or to be eligible for public office, by virtue of the fact that this certificate is issued at the time of sentence. The Date of Sentence in this case must agree with the Date Certificate Issued.

[X] b. Relieve the holder of all disabilities and bars to employment, excluding the right to be eligible for public office.

[ ] c. Relieve the holder of the forfeitures, disabilities or bars hereinafter enumerated _____

12. [X] This certificate shall be considered permanent.

[ ] This certificate shall be considered temporary until _____ After this date, unless revoked earlier by the issuing court or parole board, this certificate shall be considered permanent. A person who knowingly uses or attempts to use a revoked certificate in order to obtain or exercise any right or privilege that he would not be entitled to obtain or to exercise without valid certificate shall be guilty of a misdemeanor.

13. Signature of issuing official(s)	Print or type name(s)	14. Title(s)
[signature]	FRANCIS X. SMITH	JUSTICE SUPREME COURT

Complete the following for DCJS, only if fingerprints are not obtainable

15. Sex	16. Color	17. Height	18. Date of Birth (Month, Day, Year)
[ ] Male [ ] Female		ft. in.	

Form DP-53 (Rev. 9/72)

Chapter Nine
STANDING ORDERS

In the 1970s Emergency Medical Services (EMS) was in its infancy.

If you suffered major illness or injury in a city, your chances of survival were better there than anywhere else. Large hospital ERs were hotbeds of activity. The best clinicians taught the student physicians who rotated through them. Larger institutions offered physical resources and supportive services to the stricken as well. You had access to experience.

Whatever competence was evident in the larger institutions' ERs was a result of adaptation rather than design. Most medical schools only had a relatively brief section of their curricula dedicated to handling emergency medical or traumatic problems. Emergency-related material was a footnote to prepare the intern for a brief rotation through the ER to fulfill requirements. There was no career path in emergency medicine.

The first official training program for emergency medicine for MDs did not take place until 1970. Emergency Medicine did not become a specialty until 1979. It was essentially a brand new field trying to define itself at the same time the paramedic system was finding its way!

Small town hospital emergency rooms had the disadvantage of low volumes of traffic coupled with reliance on local physicians who were oriented to run-of-the-mill medical problems. Few, if any of the ERs were equipped with more than the essentials. They were way-stations where, theoretically, serious cases could be brought, stabilized, and then transported to a larger facility.

Local emergency systems of the day were burdened by long response times, marginal on-scene care, inexperienced ER staff, and poor communications with a proper facility, if one could even be found. There wasn't a strong web of support for the critically ill or injured.

Around the same time, however, society was moving away from the extended family into nuclear families. Fewer illnesses were being managed by relatives. Family physicians, out of self-defense from the increased workload, consolidated and moved to fill new hospitals. More people needing medical care began to be brought to emergency rooms.

This increased the volume of traffic for smaller hospitals and emergency services expanded. Unusual, complicated or horrendous cases were still treated by a cast of local physicians whose areas of expertise were predominately in routine rather than acute and/or critical problems.

Many hospitals, in order to maintain certification or be eligible for funding, were required to keep their emergency rooms open 24/7. There was little regulation of the quality of personnel who staffed them.

For a small hospital, to be a part of a paramedic program meant it would get a significant boost in status and prestige. Being designated as a paramedic base station attracted funding for upgraded facilities, and, of course, they wanted to improve their ability to serve. Because of this, many smaller facilities clamored to be a part of the program.

It only took one doctor to spearhead a movement to bring paramedic services to the local hospital. Taking advantage of the glut of funding opportunities springing up, one could manage to raise the cash to buy the base station's equipment and get money pledged to upgrade the local ambulance provider. He could then hand-pick the medics who would be trained. He would be expected to work with the county on protocols and train ER staff in the use of radio and telemetry. In a matter of six months, the new paramedic program could be staffed and rolling.

But that didn't mean the hospital was ready.

Many of the smaller hospitals had half-baked emergency services. Some only required a nurse on duty. When an emergency came in, she (few *male* nurses then) would page, or go through the switchboard to find a doctor in the house. It was a crapshoot who would be there and what they could do, or even *if they were willing!* The next step would be to call in a doctor from home. Many hospitals had an on-call system, and they were not always maintained properly. Often there were huge time lags before the physician would appear at the ER.

In 1966, as a fifteen year-old living on Long Island, I was riding in the back of a Jeep that hit a 15 ton truck head-on. I seriously dislocated my shoulder. It took over 1 ½ hours for an ambulance to get to the scene (community volunteers, converted hearse), ½ hour to get to the hospital, and another 3 hours before a Doctor presented himself.

For hospitals requiring full-time physician staffing, it was a matter of making sure a warm body was on duty. A common practice of many hospitals was to assign local physicians who were under review for misconduct, incompetence, suspension of insurance and the like to emergency service only. They would be given duty in the ER so they were not deprived of a source of income while facing their challenges. Some of these physicians included active alcoholics or drug users and the aging or even infirm who, phasing out of their own private practices, would opt for the "quieter" world of the emergency room.

So, while one or two doctors in a small hospital could be dedicated to improving emergency services and building a viable paramedic program, emerging medics would often end up spending most of their on-duty time under the direction of, let's just say, less than desirable mentors whose commitment to the program was overshadowed by their need for their own survival.

In the early years, the contrast between new, aggressive doctors and those doing time in the ERs was enough to drive a conscientious medic berserk. You could have the same exact patient, with the same exact diagnosis and the same exact symptoms two weeks in a row, and be given two completely different sets of orders — one of which would leave the patient in worse shape than when you first arrived on the scene!

For the longest time, it was up to the individual physician's discretion whether anything would be done at all with a patient. A medic could call in and present a concise, accurate report that under normal circumstances would merit a few complex treatments that were usually successful and still be told to "Get the patient in here! No orders."

Many older ER docs were resistant to people younger than themselves (especially without an MD behind their names) doing in the field what they, themselves, were reluctant or scared to do in the hospital. The medics tolerated them until they dropped out of emergency services and were replaced by more gung-ho doctors.

The proportion of doctors in ERs who chose emergency medicine as a specialty did increase. This new breed didn't proliferate until the mid 1980's. So by the time many ER physicians started working they found themselves dealing with paramedics with years more practical experience in handling emergencies than themselves.

This didn't seem to pose a problem. Most ambulance personnel at the time came up from the ranks, so many were not much different in age from the newly emerging ER doctors. Both the medics and the docs were defining new, related professions and learning about the limits and boundaries of what they were doing. It was fun and they liked the idea they were making a difference and they could make a difference together.

Newly emerging ER doctors were well-trained. Medics knew who was Boss. It felt like camaraderie with them based on building mutual respect. With the "old breed" it felt like a clashing of egos. It was the difference between "Let's try this!" and "It's God's will!"

Some medics received approval from their physicians to render advanced care to a certain level before calling in. They negotiated to find what was okay with the doctor and not. The doctor's confidence in the medic determined the complexity of the therapies allowed.

Medics tested the limits and boundaries of each doctor they worked under, always seeking to get permission to use the "next" stage of treatment in the field rather than waiting for the hospital. In a way, it was getting the system used to relying more and more on what the medics could do in the field. And then again, some of it was ego.

Each hospital had its own protocols. Theoretically medics were only to begin advanced treatment — each stage of it — *after* the doctor ordered it. Privately, doctors would tell the medics whom they trusted to follow through with their own best judgment and call in at the point at which more advanced orders were to be requested.

For protocol's sake, the medic called in and acted as if he were not taking action until orders were given, when in reality, he had done as much as he knew to do *prior* to picking up the hand-set. The doctors, and usually the rest of the ER staff as well, played along.

They knew full well it wasn't humanly possible for a medic to call in at 2:03 p.m., ask for orders to intubate, start a D5W IV, administer a 50 c.c. bolus of sodium bicarb and 5 c.c. of epinephrine, defibrillate, and then, at 2:05 p.m. call back to say "therapies were administered, defibrillation was successful and here's a rhythm strip to prove it!"

Many systems learned to trust their medics and started to grant a certain degree of formal autonomy to them. This came in the shape of "standing orders" — hospital or system-wide parameters for therapy that could be initiated by the paramedic without having to call in first.

Protocols were developed for each class and many subclasses of medical or traumatic emergencies. "Decision trees" were published wherein if "A" happens *after* "B"; follow with treatment "A6 through 10" and so on. Once the medic assessed the patient, he or she could begin therapy immediately. This showed a tremendous amount of faith in the paramedics who had worked so hard and so long for the right.

Emergency room physicians of today have had extensive training in all aspects of their specialty. The medic's role, as their eyes, ears and hands has expanded as well. Standing orders are a reflection of that mutuality. In the beginning, however, even though each doctor had to rotate through an ER during residency, once out in practice very few could or would choose to keep up with their emergency skills.

Just as medics had to prove themselves to doctors with whom they worked, so too did doctors have to pass muster with them.

"Thank God, it's Sunday..." Erin said. She had just called in to Goleta Valley Hospital for a routine beginning of shift, radio check.

"...Dr. Palumbo's on. This doesn't make me happy,"

Erin closed up the radio and checked to see there was extra rhythm strip paper for the cardiac monitor.

"Christ, another day with Dino." I said, continuing inventory.

We called him "Dino," for dinosaur. He was a throwback to the days of load and go. Whereas, by this time, 90 per cent of the ER physicians had become accustomed to and even enthused by the paramedic program, Dino refused to shift his non-cooperative stance. This was in the mid-eighties; Dino would fit well in ERs I had worked out of in Florida, back in the mid-seventies!

It may have had to do with fear of liability. He had faced a number of malpractice lawsuits in the past and didn't want to get nailed for something a medic did in his name. He was an insecure guy looking over his shoulder to see what was gaining on him and ready to snap at anything he felt threatened by. He'd report for his shift and do his work and rarely give more than basic orders.

Dino was an on-call substitute for regularly scheduled doctors who called in sick. He worked at all three local hospitals and could pop up anywhere, at any time. Because of him a lot of us started our day asking who the doctor was on duty during radio checks. When we found Dino was on, we manipulated the universe in any way we could to avoid that particular emergency room.

"What's going to happen when standing orders get approved? He gonna quit?" I wondered aloud.

"Doubtful," Erin replied, "then the County will be carrying the responsibility. He sure won't go beyond the basics still, I bet."

It did look like the county's legal department was going to approve a county-wide standing orders policy. Santa Barbara County was at the forefront of pre-hospital emergency services in the state.

The paramedic system had evolved significantly. Immediate treatments had been mapped out for many life-threatening conditions. Once the signs and symptoms corresponded with the profile of the condition, we could begin the pre-determined therapies. We had to document, of course, and make certain what we said was there was there. Then, we'd call in, report what we saw and what had been done and either await further orders or request them.

It was a lot different with Dino. He did not acknowledge standing orders. With him, we had to wait even while we knew fully what was necessary. Sometimes he'd look up what to do in a protocol book. Sometimes he'd consult with a nurse. Other times, he'd just say, "Transport." Suggesting what was needed to be done was flirting with rage. It wasn't fun to have the patient's loved ones listening to you being accused of incompetence over the radio!

Moments in the Death of a Flesh Mechanic...a healer's rebirth

Erin and I had been working in the field long enough to have used most every routine to sidestep the excruciating wait for orders that was part and parcel of working with doctors like Dino. Later that day, we sat in the living room of the one-bedroom apartment that was the town of Goleta's headquarters, and discussed sound medical strategy.

"You used the "Bad Radio" bit lately?" I asked her.

"For a diabetic; what a blast!" she said sarcastically. "I had everything done; IV in, bloods drawn, glucose administered, Everything! I expected to call in and report. Who should answer the phone but Dino. I about shit! So I gave a full report on the patient's condition, and he says, 'Start an IV of D5W.' I say, '10-4, will report back when done.'"

"He actually ordered an IV?" I said, "Wow!"

"You're right!" Erin sneered, "I just don't give that guy enough credit, do I? Anyhow, the patient is already waking up from what I did before I called in! While the fireguys are loading him into the unit, I take the radio into the bathroom and sit on the bowl. I wait a minute, 'Doctor, the IV's going; how do you feel about us drawing bloods and giving some glucose?' He goes, 'Well...' I hear the nurse in the background going 'Yes, it's protocol, Doctor. Draw bloods, administer Glucose.'"

"He pauses." Erin squints her eyes and points to her forehead. "I can tell he's really stretching his little pea brain. Then he goes, 'Draw bloods. *We'll* administer the glucose once you bring the patient here.'"

"Oh, God!" I moaned.

"What's worse is one of the fireguys comes in looking for me," she continued. "He starts yelling out my name, 'Erin, we're ready to roll!' and I know Dino can hear it. So I quick get up, open the bowl, stick the phone down into it and flush as I call out, 'Real bad radio interference, St. Francis Base. I copy draw bloods and administer 50 c.c. bolus of dextrose; will call in on the way.' Then I cut the radio."

"What happened when you got in?" I asked.

"He wrote up an incident report, of course." She laughed and then snorted. "But catch this...he wrote up the *company* for having poor gear, and he *demanded* all our radios be retested by the manufacturer!"

I liked Erin. She was as gloriously twisted as any male medic I had ever worked with; as twisted as any person I had known

The day was a blessing; nothing but two move-ups to cover the city and Goleta while the Santa Barbara units were busy with calls. The rest of the day was in front of the TV, eating, or swapping war stories. I couldn't ask for a better Sunday than to be hanging out with a very sharp, gorgeous woman who had a sense of humor that could melt granite.

My girlfriend didn't like the idea, of course. And I suppose Erin's husband wasn't crazy about it either. Here we were, a guy and a girl, sleeping in the same room (though separate beds) and living together for 48 hours on and 48 hours off. It was an ideal relationship!

All we had to do was "be" until a call came up. Then it was "be responsible together" for a half hour or so. Then hang out together; a far cry from worrying about the phone and electric bills, figuring how to talk the kids into wearing Sears's jeans instead of Designer's at three times the cost, and planning a day around a visit from mother-in-law.

We also shared intimate experiences under the category; "No one else but you could really understand."

One night we were called to respond with County Fire to a blaze. Two other ambulances were dispatched, so we expected action. We were faced with some of the thickest fog I had ever encountered. Visibility was way low. We were the closest unit to the scene.

Erin drove, and the various lights fading in and fading out and undulating and reflecting off the fog made everything feel like, we agreed, we were in the midst of an acid trip. Erin didn't dare to go faster than about 20 miles an hour. I strained my watchdog eyes to make sure we didn't run into another ambulance or fire truck also responding.

Turning on to a cross street near our destination, ahead, in the middle of the road, was a thick, gray slab of fog that looked as if it had been partially dyed with bright orange, red and yellow. It was quivering! There were two fire engines dousing it with water, sending gray black billows of steam and smoke up to the ceiling of fog that flattened out and spread like a shroud above us. There was some sort of a shape in the middle of the intertwining colors, but we couldn't identify it.

We came to a stopped Chevrolet sedan; yellow light bar on its roof flashing out caution. A squad car was next to it. A policeman and a man in coveralls were standing by it. The officer motioned us to park behind them. We got out and went to the men.

My eyes kept seeing a framework underneath the swirls, and it seemed to have windows and a tower of some sort. In its lower, left corner, there was a particularly thick blaze congregating around what looked to be a dark square. To me, it looked as if there were a house on fire underneath all that fog. But we were dead center in an intersection of two four-lane roads. It didn't make sense.

The officer described what was going on. There *was* a house on fire in the middle of the intersection. It was the top section of a two-story Victorian home. It was being towed to a new location.

"God knows why in this fog." the officer said, "an idiot in a van came flying up behind the safety car. Blew his horn like a madman..."

Moments in the Death of a Flesh Mechanic...a healer's rebirth

"He yelled out laughing, 'Get fucked, slowpoke!' as he passed me," interjected the guy in coveralls. "Had to been happy-drunk."

"...and then," the officer continued, "the van plowed right through the fog and into the corner of the house! The van blew; then, everything went up."

We were advised there was no one injured except the driver, whom the fire guys declared "Burned to death beyond repair, no doubt, can't even touch him!" we canceled the other units and went to look.

Almost casually, we sauntered up closer to the edge of the house and the van. It felt as if we were in tune, both silent and taking in the spectacle, like it was a romantic walk on the beach at twilight.

And then, as we got closer, Erin turned to me and asked, "Are we seeing the same thing here?"

Erin had words. I was speechless. I took in the whole scene.

The impact had been so great the front of the passenger side of the van was almost touching its front seat. The driver's side was thrust forward. The driver's body was partially squeezed out the open window.

The man was completely charred black like a burnt log. A two-inch deep, eight inch long crack in the crust on the body's upper left shoulder revealed a stripe of pink flesh still bubbling fluid from the heat! The rest of the body was steaming from the Fire Department's water.

I've seen "Crispy Critters" like this before, but this one was for the books! He was sitting upright in the seat and still holding his arm out the window, bent at the elbow, middle finger pointing heavenward, *shooting the bird for all eternity at the Chevy he had just passed!*

Some would say a moment shared like this is better than sex. Well, it was certainly as good as I was going to get from Erin, anyway.

At about 2:00 a.m. we were toned out for a "Man down; Santa Barbara Airport; outside the terminal." Very unusual; the airport, although servicing national flights by major airlines was pretty much shut down by midnight. Private pilots did not even use the terminal.

"Think it's a bogey?" Erin asked as she swung her legs over the side of her bed, opposite me.

"Dunno," was my intelligent reply.

I crooked an eye open and squinted to see what I could see. Too late. She clicked on the light as she stood and pulled on her jumpsuit over her stretched, non-transparent undershirt. Working with women medics sure accelerated the awakening-and-becoming-alert process!

The airport, three minutes away from our quarters, is built on a wide expanse of sand and marsh between the small town center of Goleta and the University of California, near the Pacific coast. As we pulled up in front of the terminal, we were surprised to see perhaps 50 people milling about outside. I followed the direction of their stares to the side, where, near one of the baggage collection centers there was a small clot of people in a circle on their knees.

That's the best way to find out where there's trouble in a crowd. Don't look for it; look where everyone else is looking. Erin parked the unit. I jumped out, opened the side door and grabbed the drug box and airway box. Erin followed with the radio and our baby, our Lifepak 5™.

As I made for the circle of people, a woman came up to me and said, "There's a doctor here. He's working on the poor man."

When I heard that, what I saw didn't surprise me. A man was spread flat out on the pavement, apparently unconscious. Another man was leaning over him and giving him mouth-to-mouth respirations, but because he hadn't opened the airway properly by positioning the head and neck, great loud farting sounds were coming out of the stricken man's mouth! The caregiver kept moving himself around the unconscious man, as if his own position was the cause of the problem.

At the same time as I gently put my hand on the man's shoulder and said, "Paramedic, doctor; I can take that over if you like," a fire truck pulled up to us followed by about five taxicabs.

With a relieved look on his face the man said, "That'd be best" and made room. He positioned himself right behind me, and began watching over my shoulder. I knelt down beside the fallen man and repositioned his head and gave him a couple of deep, quick breaths. Just as I felt for a pulse and found none, two firemen came up. They went to work and began two-man CPR.

I got up to step back and help Erin set up and noticed two things: One was that the taxicabs were shoveling people and their baggage in to the cars left and right and then taking off like streaks. The second was that the doctor was frozen in position, pale as a sheet and nervously wringing his fingers through his hair as he stared at the fallen man being attended to by the firemen.

On one level, he was really in the way, but then again, professional courtesy could go a long way. Some day I might need that relationship. And then, Erin and I looked at each other, and both knew we were thinking the same thing, "Screw Dino; we've got a Doc on the scene!" We both focused on setting out our equipment. Erin set up to cover the airway, while I put conductive gel on the defibrillator paddles.

"We were delayed from Denver," the doctor talked, working to calm himself, "then, when we got home — here — the tower had us in a holding pattern for about an hour, waiting for the fog to lift."

Out of the corner of my eye, I noticed fewer taxis. The ones that remained were surrounded by cadres of weary, impatient travelers.

"This guy was sitting next to me, happy to have a few more drinks while we waited," the doctor continued. "When we landed, he ran to the phone to call a cab and then...he just collapsed."

He was looking at us imploringly, as if to say, "It all happened so fast, I didn't know what to do!"

"Don't worry about it," I said. "We can use help here, though."

I motioned him over with me. Erin had just placed an endotracheal tube in the man and was withdrawing the flexible metal stylette from the tube. I worked my way in between her and the firemen, who had already ripped open the man's shirt. I put the paddles on his chest and looked at the monitor.

"He's still fibrillating, doc," I said. "How about 360 joules."

The high-pitched squeal of the charger got even more pointed. The paddles were ready. I looked around to make sure no one was touching the man, shouted out "Clear!" and hit the buttons.

The man jerked off the ground. The line on the monitor shot off the screen and then came back in very wide, irregular waves. A quick check of the pulse (none), and the firemen resumed doing CPR

Erin slapped a tourniquet around the man's arm and in a flash, got an IV started and running.

"An amp of Bicarb..." I called out while Erin already started to administer the drug, "...and 5 c.c. of Epi, what do you think, doc?"

For a second, the doctor looked startled. Then he just looked at me and shook his head yes.

Erin called out, "Bicarb and Epi on board. Still in fib! Again?" and before the doctor could even shrug his shoulders, I motioned the firemen back, and hit the buttons again. The man hopped, and this time, a very slow rhythm came across the scope.

"We've got a pulse; weak, but there." Erin had her fingers on the man's carotid artery on his neck.

Now, the doctor suddenly became excited. He leaned in toward us and the patient, and concentrated on what was going on.

A real slow sinus now," Erin spoke to the doctor as she looked at the monitor and smiled. "What do you think about some atropine?"

The doctor said, "Speed up the heart; Sure!"

I administered the atropine, while Erin put a blood-pressure cuff around the man's arm.

The monitor showed that the stricken man's heart rhythm was tightening up. His beats were coming more rapidly and regularly.

"We've got a pressure," Erin called out; "let's move!"

The doctor, the firemen, Erin and I gathered up the equipment, transferred the patient on to our gurney and into the ambulance.

One of the firemen got behind the wheel of the ambulance while Erin, me and the doctor got in the back of the unit with the patient. As the doctor stepped in, he was beaming from ear to ear.

The fireman made radio contact with dispatch just before pulling away from the terminal. He explained we had run a successful code, a local doctor was on board, and that we were on our way to the hospital with our patient.

I noticed the taxi cabs were gone, but there were a few unmarked cars that had pulled up to the terminal in the taxicab slots. The drivers were furtively looking over their shoulders as they grabbed cash out of the hands of the remaining clamoring airline passengers and then hustled them quickly into the cars. These were "Pirates"; unlicensed cab drivers who swooped in and "stole" passengers on super busy nights. A couple of the "cabs" were stuck behind us.

While Erin continued ventilating (WHOOOSH) the patient and kept her eye on the cardiac monitor, a light went off in my head. I dialed in the hospital as I turned to the doctor sitting beside me.

"Doctor (WHOOOSH), do you have privileges at Goleta Valley Hospital?" I asked.

"Goleta Base, Doctor Palumbo speaking," squawked the radio (WHOOOSH).

"Stand by a sec," I requested.

"Privileges?" the doctor replied. He really looked confused.

"Yes, sir; Privileges." I spoke so very slowly and cautiously (WHOOOSH). I felt a queasy knot moving in my belly.

"That way we can bypass the emergency room completely and admit the man, as your patient, directly into the Cardiac Care Unit."

"Oh, no..." The doctor chuckled (WHOOOSH).

"Medic Five, come in please. I'm waiting." Doctor Palumbo, on the radio, was getting angry.

"Doctor Palumbo," I waved the doctor to wait a second while I spoke into the handset, "we're en route to your facility with an (WHOOOSH) about 60 year-old man who was in cardiac arrest..."

"I'm not..." said the doctor beside me.

Before he could finish interrupting me, something clicked.

I looked at Erin and knew we were on the same page. I twisted a dial on the radio and switched off the transceiver. She nodded.

Moments in the Death of a Flesh Mechanic...a healer's rebirth

"I mean, I am a doctor...but I'm...I'm only a veterinarian...I mean, *not only*, but..." The doctor shook his head, not sure whether to be ashamed or not.

I swallowed hard; gulped was more like it. I dialed in and toned out the hospital again. Dr. Palumbo picked the call right up. I looked over at Erin. She was frozen in her tracks.

"Palumbo here. Apparently your company hasn't done anything to rectify the radio problems. I spoke with your dispatch. Just bring the patient directly to CCU. Can you copy Medic Five?"

Erin sighed in relief and snapped back (WHOOOSH WHOOOSH! WHOOOSH!!) into action.

"Five copys," I replied and cut the radio off again.

I looked at my partner and wondered which of our own hearts was about to stop first? Palumbo would be the kind of guy who'd try to nail us. He didn't like us because we didn't like him. But, God was with everybody who was in the back of the ambulance that night.

The patient started moving by the time we backed up to the hospital bay. He was even fighting having the endotracheal tube in; a very good sign.

In the CCU, our good doctor from the scene, now identifying himself as Dr. Mulholland, asked us, "Did we, um, practice medicine without a license?"

I didn't know what to say, though I didn't want to lie. So, I didn't. "Well, it seems we just saved a life, doctor," was my response.

Dr. Unger, a cardiologist, came to the nurse's station from another CCU patient's cubicle.

Erin went to Unger and grabbed him by the arm and started to speak low and conspiratorially with him. She giggled. He laughed aloud. He put one hand on her shoulder and looked at his watch. He looked at me and guffawed.

Then he turned to the nurse behind the desk.

"I'll be admitting this man," he said.

Erin and I dropped off Dr. Mulholland at home, after we went back to the airport and picked up his luggage, saving him the cab fare. It was very late.

Back at the ambulance quarters, as we got ready to go to sleep, Erin sat at the edge of her bed, clipping her fingernails.

"I feel a little dippy." she said.

"How so?" I asked.

"I actually turned on the charm to get Unger to bail us out." She laughed. "I know he's got the hots for me."

"Do you cease to be a woman, just 'cause you're a medic?" Truth was I wasn't clear on how all that worked for her.

"No, and that's the problem," she replied. "I liked it. It was fun. I knew I had him."

"So, what're you worried about?" I said. "He'll figure you want to sleep with him and then call in payback. You say 'No!' What's he gonna do?"

"It's just..." She ignored me. "Is any tool a good tool?"

Something about the way she asked prevented me from automatically responding,

"Whatever works," I said, tentatively, "...mostly..." Then I put my head under the covers and drifted off into sleep.

Chapter Ten
SUSPENDED

Hope Ranch is prime rolling countryside that provides the discerning home buyer a plethora of choices. All it costs is money, and tons of it at that, but Lord! What you can buy with it!

No parcels are smaller than a few acres. No house is valued less than a few million. Situated five minutes away from the highway or a major shopping center, for the right price, here are some of your choices:

You can live in a valley, atop a high desert hill, on a golf course, a boulevard flanked by palm trees, or on a lagoon. You can be nestled in the middle of woods with a creek gurgling below you. You can live on the ocean, or overlook the ocean from a cliff. You can have a spectacular view of the foothills and the Santa Ynez Mountains. You can overlook the city of Santa Barbara and watch it spread out toward the Pacific. In some of the locations, you can combine almost any of the above.

All this is within the radius of about a mile and a half.

Your children can go to school and board and ride horses there. All houses are connected to bridle paths. If you don't have a tennis court, there are plenty around. A pool is a given. The kids can even drunkenly race the Mercedes you bought them through the winding, dipping hills and get caught by the roving Hope Ranch Patrol and then be let off with nothing more than the threat of you, their parent, being notified.

Montecito, Santa Barbara's other plush enclave at the time, housed the "Old Rich" meaning the establishment rich, like icons Robert Mitchum and Jonathan Winters, and those with lineage such as Michael Douglas. Hope Ranch, however, was playing host to the "New Rich," people who were just now making money, lots of it, in LA, or elsewhere.

Rockers like Joe Walsh and Jackson Brown, stars like Steve Martin, and a slew of high-powered moguls of commerce and industry like Fess Parker and the Khashoggi's still call Hope Ranch their base.

Base. That's the word I used, wasn't it?

The thing Montecito and Hope Ranch share is neither is populated by people who both live and work in the area. Santa Barbara is a place where more money is spent than earned. The Great Mystery!

There's something about the interiors of Hope Ranch homes. There's more room in them than ones in Montecito; modern, spacious design. Furnishings are carefully placed; each piece of furniture, knick-knack, or decoration is meant to be seen. It's not garish display; rather, each item, by its essence, commands attention and has the space to get it.

I was trying to figure why Hope Ranch homes felt so different inside from those of Montecito. My partner Eddie and I had been called to do a "courtesy assist" for a patient confined to his bed in one of the spacious homes overlooking "Laguna Blanca", Hope Ranch's ersatz lake.

We had been instructed to "follow the open doors" through the house until we encountered a nurse. Through the front door, and down a hallway that ended in three doors, we came to an opening into a long, outside corridor sheltered by an ivy-covered trellis. It connected two sections of the immaculate Spanish style, six or so bedroom home.

We passed a large, deep maroon clay urn. It looked as if it were made in the 1800's; it had a naturally weathered appearance (as if I really knew!). A few yards later, of all things, was a stack of cannon balls. Except for a few weld marks to hold them together, they looked like the genuine articles also. In what was then a three or more million-dollar home, I couldn't imagine anyone being so cheesy as to fake it.

To the right was a garden encircling a Jacuzzi that could probably hold 10 people in comfort. At the end of the corridor, and wrapping around the garden, the walkway took a sharp right turn and then proceeded another 20 or so feet. I was somewhat surprised at how self-evident the path to our destination in the house was, given the spaciousness of the property. Ahead of us and to the right there were three wooden doors evenly spaced along the walkway. The last one was open. As we turned the corner, suddenly the connection hit me.

"People in Montecito accumulate," I exclaimed. "Here in Hope Ranch, they collect!"

"Gee, Russ, that's wonderful," Eddie replied as he nonchalantly looked into the windows to his left as he passed.

I looked in, too, and saw that each set of the multi-paned, wooden framed windows, one for each door, led to a bedroom. Odd, I thought; every item in each of the rooms was placed so precisely. The only thing missing were red felt ropes suspended by stanchions across the doorways to prevent tourists from touching anything. Eddie ducked into the last, open door. I gallantly marched in behind him into a bedroom, proud of having had my theory borne out by what I was seeing.

Moments in the Death of a Flesh Mechanic...a healer's rebirth

Technically, I was off duty. My relief, who had been delayed by car trouble that morning, was waiting for me back at the quarters. This call would be over in a minute, and then, I'd be free.

Placed at the center of a bedroom, with six feet of space in any direction between it and the walls, was a large white hospital bed. The off-white stucco walls made it feel like a hospital room from the 1800s, even though modern bedside stands, a meal table, and IV poles were in it.

There was a man in the bed. He had a tube leading from his nose to a bag filled with chalky white fluid hanging on an IV pole. I heard gurgling. I started to approach him when a queasy feeling in my gut led my eyes over to the far left corner of the room. The shading there disturbed me, as if something was waiting to spring out.

Sticking out of the walls were a pair of arms and a face fringed with a half halo of hair. My eyes adjusted, and I saw a woman wearing a white nurse's uniform backed into the corner. She had a nurse's cap on her head, off center. Unkempt folds of her hair were darting out from it, suggesting she had been running her fingers through her hair.

"Thank God, you're here!" She made a beeline for the door.

"Hold on a minute." Eddie put his body between her and the door. "How about filling us in?" He wasn't making a request.

My partner had her covered. I continued to the man in the bed. My eyes zeroed on the gurgling. It was coming from his throat. Suddenly, there was only that man's airway and the gurgling; no Hope Ranch, partner or woman. Soon he would drown in his own fluids.

Just below his Adam's apple was a half-inch diameter hole with a flap of skin that bulged out from it every time he exhaled. Hanging around his neck was a gauze tie about a half-inch wide. Hanging from that was a curved metal tube three inches long and a half-inch in diameter. It was bouncing up and down on his chest like an oversized pendant as he coughed wet and ominously. That metal tube was the man's airway! It was supposed to be in that hole, and it wasn't.

His neck was hyper extended, and his lips had a tinge of blue to them. Although it appeared he had been getting air, apparently he was working on a deficit. His shoulders were tense and straining; his eyes glued to the ceiling. This man was crossing the line into crisis. There was something strange about him, too. It was as if he weren't present. Under such circumstances, I would expect him to have been looking more panicked, perhaps looking to me for help.

He'd noisily cough out and then try to take in a breath. His in-breath was a struggle, and when he actually did get some air in, it accentuated his gurgling, from more secretions. After every attempt to bring in air, he'd cough an alarming cough. But he didn't appear to be connected to the danger he was in.

Everything was a physical reaction with no underlying connection to his psyche — an almost robotic response. I started to get a clearer sense of what I was dealing with.

The metal tube hanging from the gauze around his neck was a standard, post-surgical tracheotomy tube. I looked around the bed and bed stands for the stylette — a bullet-shaped metal plug inserted into the hollow tube so it can be reinserted into the stoma, the hole in his neck.

"Here it is," Eddie called out, "She had it."

He put it in my hand. I wiped it off on the bed sheet. Gingerly untying the gauze tie around his neck and taking the tracheotomy tube in my hand, I inserted the stylette into the hollow tube.

"She's never had a patient anything like this," Eddie reported as I positioned myself. "It was just supposed to be routine nurse's aide type care. She was giving him a bed bath when she got startled and slipped and knocked it out. It freaked her. She was afraid to go near him."

I could see why. It was like being near Frankenstein's monster during a short circuit! Holding the stylette in my hand, I placed it just above the hole in the man's neck. I waited for him to take in his next breath. When he did, I carefully inserted the tube. The next, quick step was to pull the stylette out and leave the hollow tube in. I wasn't fast enough, because the second the tube was inserted, with the solid stylette blocking his air passage, he choked and gave a mighty cough and blew it out of his trachea, out of my hand and onto the floor.

It startled me so I chuckled aloud when it took off flying across the room! Eddie fetched the tube and opened one of the stands and rummaged through it. He found alcohol swabs and K-Y™ jelly, a lubricant. He disassembled and wiped off the tube with the swabs, put K-Y™ around the rim of the plug, reassembled it and handed it to me.

"Grease, Russ," Eddie said, "You forgot the grease."

Once again, I positioned myself and waited. A cough and then a breath and then another cough. On the next inhalation, the tube went in smoothly and the stylette came out just in time for the man to cough loudly. With the tube in place, the cough sounded much more clear and resonated like a blast of wind through a tunnel. A thin stream of viscous saliva expelled with the wind.

There was a suction machine by the bed, and together we pulled out thick fluid from the man's upper airway. He started breathing more easily right away. And then he slid into a vacant stare toward the wall.

A little alarmed, I waved my hand in front of him to elicit a reaction. None. Did he fry his brain just while we had been there?

"He's a head injury," Eddie said. "She says he's in a coma."

"There's two phone numbers for you here." The nurse's aide spoke, voice quivering as she moved a pad of paper over to a phone on a bureau by the door leading to the interior of the home. "The first is his relative's. The second is the doctor's." She motioned to the phone.

"I'm emergency relief; I'm leaving." She walked out the door.

Eddie and I looked at each other in surprise. "Well," Eddie said, "looks like we adopted a patient."

And what a patient this one was!

We did a head-to-toe assessment to cover our bases. Each of us took a side, and with completion of each level — head, neck, shoulders, chest, etc. — we called out "clear," or noted anything unusual. The man appeared to be in his 40s, judging by silver streaks in his blond hair. At one time, he may have been very handsome, but it was hard to tell; his face was contorted into a grimace. Clean shaven, his skin had obviously been meticulously cared for. It had a sun-deprived, pasty sheen to it. His eyes were open, but you wouldn't call him conscious. No spark.

"Everything clear; sluggish pupil. You?" I asked.

"Same," was Eddie's reply.

The head of the bed was elevated. He was being supported by it and a large pillow along each side of his torso, wedging him in between the guardrails. Thank God he was upright, I thought. Were he to have been laid flat, he for sure would have drowned in his own fluids.

His lungs were clear, his heart sounded strong and regular, and there was no sign of trauma or injury to his torso. His arms and legs, though bent at the joints, were not exactly loose, yet they were not rigidly in contracture as usually seen in elderly patients not cared for properly. They, too, were absent of injury or trauma, or even old scars.

I took a BP while Eddie checked a bedside stand to find a chart.

"I say he's been out of the hospital a couple three weeks," I offered as my conclusion. "Everything's stable here."

"Wrong, wrong, wrong," Eddie replied. "Try four years."

"Four years!" I exclaimed and then caught myself for fear of having the patient hear me.

"I guess we better call the number." Eddie picked up the phone.

It was the number of the patient's wife. Eddie explained the situation and asked her questions. No one had ever walked out on them before, she said. This was a new girl who was covering for their regular, live-in aide who was out of town for an emergency for the day. She was a friend of the family who just started working as an aide. The woman was worried that anyone new would be equally unable to handle the task.

Eddie quickly relayed the info to me. She was scheduled to come this evening, he said. Until then, she was really caught off guard.

Scheduled to come? I remembered the house didn't look lived in. The scene was befuddling me, and I wanted to understand. I got on the phone and spoke to the woman. The next thing I knew, I was volunteering to look after the man until six p.m.

"Are you nuts?" Eddie asked after I got off the phone. "You come back to work tomorrow. It's not even your three-day coming up."

"All I'll have to do is stay awake," I replied. "She said she'd pay me what I get paid for a day, so it's nine o'clock now; an extra seventy-five won't kill me." I lied. But money is usually the easiest explanation for taking on a duty that others think is strange.

It was very simple to make arrangements. First, we called the man's doctor and reported what had happened. It wasn't necessary to bring him in to be seen. "Just suction if his throat is still kicking up junk," he said. Next, we checked with dispatch to find other city units were available to cover. Eddie would put the ambulance out of service for six minutes and go back to quarters. He'd pick up my relief and be ready to run a call. The patient's wife agreed to get me a ride back to quarters and my car. It seemed like a fairly smooth transition.

Within 10 minutes, all was arranged. Eddie was gone, and I was alone with the patient. The first thing I did was go to the table that held the chart Eddie was reading. In one of its drawers was a tabbed, loose-leaf notebook filled with history. I took it, sat down, and began reading.

Peter Markle was a newly married 44-year-old owner of an upstart computer manufacturing firm in L.A. It got bought out, and his life transformed overnight. Suddenly wealthy, he and his wife moved to Hope Ranch. She had twins. (Sociological Assessment Report)

One morning, at two a.m. coming up from LA in his Mercedes sports convertible after a late Friday night business dinner and drinks, he ran off the highway, overturned the car and crashed into a ditch. Another car on the road stopped immediately, and the driver got right to him. He found Peter half in and half out of the car, legs above his head, and face down in a patch of soft dirt. His neck was hyper-flexed forward. He wasn't breathing and was unconscious. The motorist was sure he was dead. Another motorist, seeing the accident occur, drove directly to a phone and called the accident in. (CHP Accident Report)

Within six minutes of impact, a fire truck arrived. The firemen gingerly flipped him over and out of the car on to his back. According to protocol, one swept out the man's mouth first. There was a clod of dirt in it. The fireman tried mouth-to-mouth and was met by resistance.

Moments in the Death of a Flesh Mechanic...a healer's rebirth

After more attempts and sweeping, the fireman did something very bold. He took his pocket knife and carefully made an incision into Peter's throat through a palpable notch below the bulge of his Adam's apple. He then inserted the tube from his pen into it and began blowing into the opening. Technically it's called a cricothyroidotomy. The report said the fireman had never done such a procedure before. Within a few of the fireman's breaths, respiration began spontaneously. The fireman found Peter had a pulse. (Fire Department Incident Report).

By then, an ambulance arrived. Physical examination showed the only thing wrong with Peter was he had that clod of dirt in his mouth and was unconscious. Taking no chances, the medics used a scoop stretcher to pick him up and secured him to it as if he were a spinal cord injury, started an IV to keep a vein open in case of emergency, and did nothing more but carefully stabilize the pen tube. (Paramedic Report).

Considering all that could have gone wrong, Peter was lucky. But the lack of oxygen fried his brain. He never regained consciousness. At one point, they said he was in a "waking coma," but by the end of the Neurological Report, even that cheery description had been abandoned.

After two months in hospital and another 30 days in the Santa Barbara rehabilitation facility, it was determined that future progress could be expected to be extremely limited. The odds of his regaining consciousness were "poor". (Hospital Chart and Discharge Report)

He was discharged to his home with a regimen of physical therapy, tube feeding and regular changes of position to prevent bedsores, along with maintenance of the stoma. This was to be his life. (Home Health Care Plan).

With the exception of three hospital visits after his discharge, one for a change in diet and two more for respiratory problems, that room had been his home for the last three years and nine months.

After more than a year and a half of doing the best she could, his wife decided to move out of the house but not out of his life. Still dedicated to Peter, she visited at least four times a week. Yet she was determined to move on with her life and provide a good environment for the children. For her, the buffer of distance would be enough.

Luckily, there were more than enough investments, and insurance from the company. Special provisions had been made to assure his, hers and the kids' future. She was able to buy another home only a few minutes away. (Sociologist's Follow-up Report)

All this from a three-ring binder!

Medical and sociological curiosity was not exactly my reason for staying at the house. Here was a man who had lost it all in less than 10 minutes. I had patients who had similar things happen to them, but never anyone who had survived so long. In one year in Santa Maria, I stabilized five gunshot wounds to the head. Bookends all, yet, each died within 30 days at most. There had to be a reason. There had to be something that made Peter different.

So I sat with Peter Markle, and walked around, touched and explored him and thought about him for close to five hours. I opened myself to feel his presence. If there was something, I wanted to feel it.

This was not something out of my character. Someone who hasn't been there may think it a bit odd — maudlin. But to me, it made sense. I wanted to know what could be the results of my own handiwork when carried to the extreme. What happens four years after a life is plucked from death, yet death refuses to release its grip? What is *alive*?

My first time alone with a dead body was a similar experience. I was 18 and working in a nursing home. A woman in her 80s came in five days earlier, lucid as could be. What she lucidly knew was that a nursing home was the last stop and that must mean her, too.

As she was admitted, she kept saying, incredulously, "This is where people come to die!" Naturally, the staff told her not to be ridiculous. Without anything serious wrong with her, she became withdrawn and silent, and within five days, she willed herself to death.

A rookie nurse's aide on the floor, I was tossed a plastic bag with everything needed to prepare it for the funeral home.

It: Now it was an "it" where once it had been a woman. How strange. Why was that?

There were other things I wanted to know. I wanted to experience certain words; certain expressions, like "Cold as death"; "Dead weight"; "A stiff"; "Death rattle"; "Rigor mortis"; "Give up the ghost"; "Lose one's life"; "Cold and clammy"; and "Shit-eating grin."

One by one, I said the expression to myself and moved my hands to touch, ears to listen, or eyes to see. I spent a half hour doing nothing but examining this woman who a little while ago had been brave enough to call a spade a spade, and then made her last choice on this planet, which was to follow through on her assessment of the situation.

I couldn't help admire her choice. I wrote a poem about the experience:

There are things you do to a life that's all through

before the mortician practices his art.

There are techniques you can master to help it

go faster, but the basics come first, so let's start.

Closing the eyes is no easy task; the reason it's done?

To help your *own* fears pass! You'll get them closed

Moments in the Death of a Flesh Mechanic…a healer's rebirth

once; they'll open again. So you try three more times!
Then you just let them stand.

Around the loose, open jaw a gauze ribbon is tied tight,
so it won't get stuck open when rigor mortis does bite.
The first thing done when baby begins life's grind, is
the last thing done, too. It's to wipe the behind.

(For so long, things were kept inside, closed.
On the way out this door; everything gets let go.)

Arms and legs must not flail and flop all around
so they get laced together, immovably bound.
The last thing done, before the covering is applied,
is the part that assures the body is shipped right.

A little tag is filled out; it says who, where and what.
To the big toe it's tied, with a real secure knot.
Then a big plastic sheet is folded over just so,
and the body is wrapped in a package to go.

But before it's shipped off, a detail at all cost: The
big toe and tag are *exposed* so the bod won't get lost.

So thanks! Mrs. Tomblin for the lesson learned today,
'cause now I know how to send someone on their way.
I know it meant something, as impersonal as it seemed;
my only hope is I'll sleep, and not see you in my dreams.

Now, 15 years after that exploration, I found myself feeling the same curiosity and wonder at what was happening. Here, with someone suspended between life and death, I had to know what was left.

He had so much movement! He blinked, furrowed his brow, twisted his face into a sneer, sneezed, chewed, twitched his eyebrows, closed one or both eyes, wrinkled his nose, coughed, opened and closed his hands, moved arms and legs (albeit minimally), yet none seemed to be a response to a stimulus. There was no spark in his eyes to hint at any conscious connection with anything. Yet, there were times he closed his eyes and I could have sworn he was sleeping as well.

It was as if there was an old tape of moments of movements playing somewhere that would suddenly and randomly scan and play and then shut down. As if groups of his muscle cells would remember, "Hey, we used to do that" and then do that. But the follow-through would be in grimacing slow motion, and never from cause and effect.

The physical aspect — how he behaved — was not as important to me as was the chance to be around him and feel what I felt. The binder gave me all the details I needed. What remained was to grasp what this human had become.

Somewhere there is a fireman who brags, humbly admits, or combining them, simply says that he saved this man's life. Regardless of how he handles it, he deserves to have his pride; for this life seemed to be slated to go, and now it remains.

There's a good chance that, in the fireman's eyes, Peter Markle is still whole. That's the way it is; you do the work, breathing gets restored, the heart returns. The patient is young and you're victorious; a clean save! Why would you possibly seek to find out otherwise?

It is a beautiful assumption to believe your labors have paid off in a life restored. I did some mental arithmetic. Over the course of my experience, how many lives had I saved and then pictured as having futures? Thirty? How many of them did I know for sure? Two perhaps.

For how many of the rest had I actually been the agent of one, two or 20 years of hell for their families? I was aware of six patients who stayed alive in comas for a month or so. But years? Considering most of my work was done in towns where local hospitals would automatically transfer severe cases to regional medical centers, there was no way I'd know. There could be many.

I checked my watch to see it was time to reposition Peter in the bed. This was an every-two-hour routine. It was essential to keep his weight off of his bony prominences, like hips, elbows, knees, and sacrum. If not, pressure of bone on flesh on bed could easily result in a decubitus ulcer — a bed sore. It starts as a small, almost imperceptible redness, and progresses until it's a gaping hole in the flesh; an easy portal through which infection can pass. People die from bedsores. That was the case with Christopher Reeve, of *Superman* fame.

I lowered the head of the bed, laid him on his other side and then raised it partially again. My work was done for that phase.

Moments in the Death of a Flesh Mechanic...a healer's rebirth

I went back to the binder and Peter's chart. For his first month post-accident, Peter's grasp on life had been maintained by around the clock, heroic efforts. Physiologically, he short-circuited. Raging fevers, lung-collapsing coughs, pneumonia, staph infections, traveling blood clots from improper circulation in his extremities, heart dysrhythmias, and intestinal stasis all dogged him unmercifully during that time.

At first, the doctors could not provide a firm enough prognosis to help the family decide whether pulling the plug was an option. Then, Peter's body started going through one crisis after another. Before the medical staff realized it, they were locked in a day-to-day struggle putting out fires. Peter had become a technical challenge. Any one of the conditions could have been the last straw. But medical knowledge had grown so each problem was correctable; an antibiotic here, a temporary colostomy there, steroids, blood thinners, heart blockers, chest tubes, each judiciously applied at the right time, kept him going.

Peter's body happened upon a sequence of ailments that, alone or in combination, were not enough to do him in. He was still young and strong enough to resist every punch. Then, the juggling act was over; the crises passed. Enough time had been bought so Peter's body found some equilibrium. Unfortunately, it was without what we identify as his mind.

Peter was a casualty of a technological drive that surpassed his body's best efforts to end its journey. Even as little as two years earlier, he never would have survived. In fact, had the accident occurred a mere five miles farther away from the fire station, it would all have been over.

Peter Markel as he sat before me four years post-injury was basically a reflection of man's headlong quest to beat death.

Every species strives to become immortal. Evolution theory tells us that. One by one, every characteristic that hastens death, or makes the species vulnerable, is being discarded in favor of a factor or two that, when passed on, will allow the next generation to live just a bit longer.

Nature seems to be content with the pace at which this marvel unfolds. That is, of course, with the exception of humankind. For some reason, we do our best to accelerate the process — no matter how much pain or death is caused in the doing. Peter serves as an example of technology triumphing over mechanical failure. But in the development of each process that extended Peter's life one more day, how many lives had been sacrificed while the bugs were being worked out?

Every time a new drug appears for use in emergencies, the same thing happens. Physicians use it. They find it drops the blood pressure when another drug like it is on board. They give a drug to raise the blood pressure, and that, with the others, speeds the heart to an alarming rate. They treat that. It goes on and on like a juggling act of which one item is a meat cleaver. They lose patients, but in the process learn the proper sequence. Peter had received the benefit of all that juggling and all the death and debility that had gone with it through trial and error.

Isn't that the way of life? It's not one sperm cell that bravely penetrates the ovum and fertilizes it; it's *millions* of sperm cells who beat their heads literally to death against the cell wall of the ovum until one tiny spot of it is ruptured enough to allow the entry of *The One*.

In rehabs and nursing homes and intensive care units throughout the globe, cardiac cripples, the brain-dead and the stroked-out live on in their own private purgatories, limbos and hells. It's not a plague quite yet, but I'll tell you this, it's moving in that direction.

What I witnessed was a society unwilling to share in the responsibility of caring for its aged infirm. Precious cargo was entrusted to mercenaries. That hasn't changed. The upcoming slide into oblivion of my generation, the Baby Boomers, is not a pretty picture to anticipate. We have learned to preserve life without promoting living. The future promises more of the same. The only difference is there will be many more of us, we'll be older, and last much longer.

Ironically, the societies most adept at destroying lives are also the most skilled at saving them. High-pressure work, affluence, alcohol, and fast cars are elements that produce head injury patients like Peter. Injuries like his have, through practice, become treatable. Sophisticated destruction walks hand-in-hand with sophisticated repair.

We are, however, making headway in our quest to beat death; witness the lengthening of the average lifespan. What we have forgotten, or deny, is limitation is incorporated into the design of all creatures great and small. Eventually, everything gives out. They say even the sun.

In a sudden outburst, Peter grimaced wildly and thrust out a fist at me. It wasn't actually aimed at me so it didn't connect. But the muscles of his arms were so intent and shaking in muscular spasm, and Peter for a moment growled like an animal so viciously, spittle flying, I jumped away from the bed; sure he was going to kill me! Then, as fast as it happened, it was over. I stood there shaking, looking at Peter in disbelief. I bet to myself that's what happened with the Aide.

Regaining my composure, I moved into Mechanic mode. I laid down the head of the bed to reposition Peter as scheduled. Remembering my old nurse's training, I reviewed the litany of maintenance guidelines the specialty of geriatric nursing had become. Double-check guardrails. See if the bowels had moved. Check the dressing on an emerging bed sore. Listen to breath sounds; make sure no suctioning was needed. I heard myself saying aloud "Don't snag the Foley catheter!" I laughed.

I was hyperaware of that Foley line; a tube passed into the bladder through the urethra and anchored by an air-expanded sleeve. It leads to a bag that collects

Moments in the Death of a Flesh Mechanic...a healer's rebirth

the patient's urine. Once, early on as an EMT, I snagged my foot in a line and tripped. I heard the "PoP!" I will never forget as the catheter ripped out of my patient's bladder! The major harm was done to me, thankfully. I hoped Peter hadn't heard my thoughts.

The bed was Peter's space capsule: His excretions were taken care of; he was well-fed via formula draining into his stomach through a tube in his nose; even a television was positioned within his sight as if a porthole. I had an urge to turn it on to see where we were both going.

What if it had been me who had kept Peter alive long enough to get into the hospital, and I had known about the aftermath? It would have taken work on my part to reconcile my role. Why? Because it looked like Peter was going to stay alive for a long time. That would have been my handiwork.

On one level, he would be sure reminder that we are triumphing over death — that I was, indeed, playing a significant role in the drama. Yet Peter himself received no benefit whatsoever from the victory. If anything at all he was an abandoned shell; and to what purpose?

Perhaps Peter was a symbol of us, Homo sapiens, pulling together our primitive resources and knowledge and pushing one of us over the top. Some day, there'd be a Peter who never died. Some day, based on what we learned from all those other Peters, there'd be someone who never died and enjoyed the trip, too!

That was the angle I needed to hold on to. My job was to bring people who were wounded as badly as Peter back — no matter what. That, I reasoned, was acting as part of a greater good. I had to be satisfied with the fact that as an individual I wasn't important. Both mine and the lives I saved were all important as reflections of a greater unfolding. Perhaps everything I did was the embodiment of that great human push toward immortality. If so, then, a lot of things made sense.

Meantime, I had to accept people like Peter would be brought back by people like me and end up just like Peter. I had no business imposing my narrow view on the world because, given a glimpse of *this*, had it been up to me, I would have said "let Peter die!" And I would have been wrong because were he not here, somehow my species would be losing ground and I wouldn't be getting the lesson.

At three p.m., a male and female team of physical therapists, Michael and Ruth, came into the room. Four days a week, they came to work with Peter for an hour and a half. I realized I was tired. I was used to working in short, intense bursts. This was living in constant watchfulness of Peter, and *me*! At any moment, I expected Peter to get up, rip the tubes out of his body, say, "Screw this; I'm leaving," and split. It had happened once before. I really wanted him to do that!

After making contact and warmly introducing themselves with a "Hi, Peter, it's us!", the physical therapists went to work stretching his arms and legs, massaging and working with every muscle group in his body. I gravitated toward a chair in the corner and sat down and watched. From the second they came into the room until the moment they left, they talked to Peter as if he were a real person. They stroked him tenderly as they told him about their lives, made comments about his wife and kids, and even shared jokes with him.

Peter, motionless except for involuntary twitches, was passive in their hands. An hour into the session, however, Michael was stretching out his right leg and out of nowhere, Peter blasted out air so forcefully some bypassed the tracheotomy and produced an ungodly raspy growl.

"Was he in pain?" I asked.

"Ask him," Ruth replied. "Don't ask us."

So I got up and asked, "Peter, are you all right?"

He looked nowhere and at nothing and smacked his lips..

"Have you been working with Peter long?" I asked Michael.

"On and off," he replied, "Both Ruth and I have for two years."

"What do you think," I stammered, "I mean...do you think he's there? That something's there?"

"Sometimes I think so," Ruth said.

"Me, too," Michael said.

"We'll never know," Ruth said. "I'd rather be wrong acting like the answer was 'Yes'".

I had nothing else to say. I took the opportunity to go to the bathroom and then get a bite to eat out of the well-stocked refrigerator. When I returned, they were getting ready to leave.

"How many patients are there like Peter here in town?" I asked. "That you take care of I mean — like this. Not sick enough to be in the hospital or rehab, confined to home, but, like a..."

I didn't want to use the word "vegetable." Michael saved me.

"Peter's one of two in the county," he replied. "The other's a teen, a head injury from a motorcycle wreck. Strokes at this level of function are usually in nursing homes."

"Peter's lucky," Ruth chimed in. "So is the other one, actually. It's the really young ones..."

"With money or from money," Michael interposed.

From money, I said to myself. That's how we think of it.

"...or with other resources," Ruth added. "They get to stay home. There's a facility down south that is a specialized head-trauma nursing home that houses quite a few like Peter. Although none of the others that we've done outcall for here have the house to themselves."

I didn't get what she meant but didn't think to question. A few minutes later, they were gone. We were alone. Peter's eyes were open.

I had a hard time looking. I was ashamed. From the moment I arrived until then, I hadn't once viewed Peter as a being. From the jump, I assumed no one was home. I buried myself in the technical problems, then in the decision to stay or not; then into alternating basic care with keeping my head in thought and buried in the binder. But, what if?

Five hours of avoidance. All my thoughts to that moment were geared toward nothing more than the flesh in front of me. Peter was an abandoned car to me, one with an interesting repair record. Yet, I couldn't connect with the mechanics of the car until I found its driver.

I went up to Peter and looked closely at him. I contrasted what I saw with what I knew of death. Peter most certainly was not dead. Death leaves a pall on the body beyond lack of movement. In *Romeo and Juliet*, Shakespeare described it well: "Death lies on her like an untimely frost upon the sweetest flower of all the field." "An untimely frost", this aspect I knew.

The part that bothered me was I could not feel presence with Peter. Again I sought the spark in his eyes that simply wasn't there. It was like looking into a bottomless well. Yet, he wasn't dead! There was animation, but no presence. Indeed, there didn't seem to be any "present" for Peter. Peter's last moments had passed four years earlier. Now, all that was left was maintaining that which stays when everything else goes.

I wondered, if deep inside... Without warning even to myself! I looked Peter right in the eyes and screamed at the top of my lungs, "Get mad, Peter! *GET MAD!!*" Nothing happened.

All I could see was a conglomeration of flesh that did all the basic things but didn't have that unifying stuff, the glue perceived as a glow that is not seen with the eyes but is felt in the heart. It is the stuff that lets you know there is another presence like yourself about. Still, that was a human being in a state that human beings can become, and that includes me! I shuddered at the challenge and dropped the thought.

I put my hands gently on his chest. Amidst the struggle, while doing CPR on a pulseless and non-breathing patient, there were times I could feel something tugging; a presence. I wanted to with Peter, but no.

"Peter," I said aloud, "I want to believe you're just sleeping."

I pulled a chair over beside him, took one of his hands in mine and sat. A wave of fear passed through me. I realized how I clung to the belief in a soul. It helped me to say even in my failures as a medic I was simply playing a part in the transition from corporeal life to eternity. But what is *this* about? I let go of the hand of a soul-less shell.

"Are you here?" I challenged him. "Or somewhere far away?"

I had to chuckle to myself at how bizarre this scene was.

"I'm still here." I said "I get to ask stupid shit." And then I stopped short, feeling guilty for bragging about the life living in me.

With the exception of his position change at about 5:30, I just sat with Peter in silence. No longer was I there to see what he had become. Rather, it was to ponder what I had, he didn't and more to the point, what I had become.

A clock in the house struck six p.m. Peter's wife came in. My relief arrived in more ways than one! She calmly stepped into the room. The first thing she did was go up to Peter and give him a big hug. She wiped his lips free of some drool and then kissed him.

"I'm here. Honey," she said; nothing from him. She came to me.

"I really appreciate you staying," she said. "These were such unusual circumstances. We stopped using people from the registries because we never knew. It's too much for some. Was it hard for you?"

I wanted to share with her the questions, the doubts; everything.

"No," I said. "It all went very smoothly. I had to dust off some old nursing skills, though."

She actually laughed. I wondered if I'd be able to do that were it my wife lying in a bed like that for four years. Of course, I would.

There was commotion in the hallway; the scampering of feet. I thought about that old pot and wondered how vulnerable it was. Two children came bursting into the room; a boy and a girl, a pair of blond, glowing twins. They exuberantly ran up to Peter's bedside and stopped.

"Mommy?" the boy asked.

Both kids stood side by side, legs bowed, blond hair flowing, leaning forward in anticipation like a British royal family portrait.

"Okay, Pete," the woman said, and the little four-year-old boy carefully turned around and went to the foot of the bed and released the latch of the guardrail. Together, he and his sister let it down. Then they went to the latch at the head of the bed and repeated the process.

Then, both of them carefully climbed up onto the bed with their father. They sat quietly with him for a moment, watching. Then, they both simultaneously gave a screech of joy and hugged him all over.

They started chattering: "Daddy, at school today, I..." "We're going to Disneyland on a church trip next..." — just like kids do with their father. The little girl brought out a crumpled, folded piece of paper from her pocket and waved it in front of Peter's face. "See what I drew for you?" She giggled.

Had not the woman motioned to me and said, "Let's leave the kids alone with him; they only get to see him a couple times a week," I may have walked away myself. I could barely watch for another second.

She ushered me out to an atrium and then to a living room. It was as clean and undisturbed as every other room I had been in.

"I'm Darla," she said as she extended her hand to me and then indicated for me to sit beside her on the couch. Of course I knew Mrs. Markle was Darla. I knew everything from that binder. I felt like a thief.

"Things are running as smoothly as can be," she said. "Just a year ago, I thought it would never, ever get back to any sort of normal."

"The kids seem to be handling it pretty well," I said. "They're really..." I grappled for a word that wouldn't reveal my hardened heart because I thought they were nuts. Giving up, I finished, "...amazing."

"I suppose they are," she replied. "It's not really a usual experience of growing up now, is it?" She laughed. "But it sure is growing up..." And then, she sighed.

"For all of you, I bet." I realized that she was only about 35.

"Yes, all of us," she answered.

Then she got up and started to tidy up some knickknacks on the shelves. I noticed she still wore her wedding ring. It had a huge diamond on it. Around her neck was a golden cross. She was an attractive young woman.

"I get to make all these corporate-sized decisions about the estate," she reflected. "It seems so odd. By day I act like an executive, and at night I take care of the kids and then go to prayer circles."

"Is that right?" I commented.

"Oh, not as much as I used to," she said. "It's different for me now. Everything is a whole lot different. I used to pray for him to wake up; to come back." Her nervous energy spent, surprisingly fast, I thought, she sat back down. She was centered again.

"But there have also been times when I haven't wanted him back," she continued. "Suddenly, his money became his life, and now I've taken over, and now it has become mine. Does that make sense?"

I nodded my head in assent.

"There was a long period of time when I was furious at God for putting us through this." Darla's eyes showed a trace of the despair. "He doesn't go. But he isn't really here; to me, anyhow."

She furrowed her brow, and her eyes became clear, determined.

"But," she went on, "I watch the children with him. He's not their toy. He's not a piece of furniture; they're not afraid, and they seem to *relate*. It's like they get to play with his spirit. Peter's not the shell."

When I got back to my car that evening, I drove myself to a movie. After the movie, I stuffed myself silly at an Italian restaurant. After that, I went home and lay in bed awake and stared at the ceiling where I replayed the scene of the children crawling around on the lap of the only father they ever knew. All I could envision was their content and connected expressions.

I mourned the loss of the part of me that once could recognize what I could not see. And when I was spent, I refused to drop into the unconsciousness of slumber.

Chapter Eleven
MEN AND MACHINES

In the field, crucial moments barrel on, one after the other, relentlessly and irreversibly. Many things occur before the delivery of advanced emergency care is even considered.

The moment you get into the ambulance, heightened awareness must snap on like an internal Klieg light. No two emergencies are alike, so there's precious little pre-planning you can do. While knowing each procedure backwards and forwards, you must be ready to think out of the box. At best, you can be sure your tools are ready and prepare yourself for the unexpected. Essentially it's about awakening the Mechanic inside.

Driving to and from the scene in practice means the only rule of the road is to respond to the moment. Yes, there are many guidelines to follow, but at all times you must remember your vehicle is in uniform. People don't know how to behave around you.

Professional race drivers say the most dangerous roadways in the world are everyday roads with everyday drivers. When the marginal attention of a driver is suddenly interrupted by the sensory explosion of lights and sirens, panic often ensues. Rather than clearing out of your way, he or she often obstructs it.

Sometimes it looks like you're breaking all the rules. But most localities have rigid guidelines that include when and how to cross a double-yellow line and enter the opposing lane of traffic for example. Behind the wheel, however, being within legal parameters is secondary to acting appropriately.

Of course, "appropriately" is a relative term. You can use a simple, mathematical formula to help you predict your chances of beating the complaint, dodging the ticket, or successfully begging the Judge to restore your Ambulance Driver's Certificate. It's based on one's experience plus skill level, minus the infraction and damage caused, divided by previous offenses, plus judgment calls (negative or positive values), plus the situation, minus the restrictions of the law and acts of God, and finally multiplied by your ability to justify your choices entertainingly minus any negative personal or professional baggage you carry squared by any formal complaints lodged against you.

Typically the *driver* drives and the *patient man* "attends" to the patient in the back. En route to the scene or hospital, the patient man navigates and acts like the "eyes in the back of his head" for the driver. Being the navigator is as important as being the driver. Most medics establish a further differentiation between the two roles when it comes to who does what during actual patient care as well.

Physical control of the scene — establishing authority, and coordinating standers-by and allied professionals such as fire and police personnel — requires diplomacy and finesse that cannot be taught by a book. There are no advanced tools to lean on. It's all about the way you carry yourself.

Information gathering, psychological support of family and friends, and evaluation of the circumstances begin as soon as the medics arrive. If you think of it as providing immediate, non-invasive care, you are on the right track. Observation, analysis, and priority setting occur before any decisions are made even remotely concerned with rendering advanced levels of care. Initially, it's all about management of the environment of the call; every aspect of it.

The logistics of the scene include identifying obstacles between you and the patient and between the patient and you. That would include the possible resistance of others who are "close to" the patient physically and/or by connection.

From the beginning, you need to identify a viable exit, activate an internal time clock that ticks away the time you have before "load and go" becomes essential, and identify who there will help and who must be moved out of the way. As time goes on, you add more items to check off on your list of "variables". Why? Because you've learned by trial and error, when you miss one, it comes back to bite you in the ass.

The cable that connects all of the above is communication. This involves partners, the patient(s), family, friends, uniformed personnel at the scene, dispatch, doctors, nurses and other allied personnel at the hospital. Mastering all of the aspects of communication is an art in itself.

These can be talked about in books or dealt with in lectures, but, when it comes to coordinating and applying them in the real world; nothing but experience that includes lots of failure will do. It boils down to being able to communicate the particulars of your immediate situation so succinctly, you can get done what you believe needs to get done.

One job description of the emergency medical technician (EMT) would be to establish and maintain control of an unpredictable environment so a patient or patients can be stabilized and safely moved. This, the most foundational aspect of the EMT's job, is often the most difficult to master.

Moments in the Death of a Flesh Mechanic...a healer's rebirth

On a non-paramedic unit, with just two EMTs, the focus is on "there": What can be done to manage this scene enough to get the patient out of here safely and to the hospital? The paramedic, on the other hand, must think in terms of "here": What can be done, right here, right now, to stabilize the patient *before* we leave for the hospital? At some point both the paramedic and EMT run into their limitations and the hospital is the *only* next step, but the EMT's limits come much earlier.

The EMT affects the patient by what can be done directly with the hands: Remove from danger; open the airway; mechanically assist circulation (CPR); stop bleeding; position; splint fractures; stabilize the spine; move; make more comfortable, and; monitor. The administration of outside agents with specific medical effects is limited to oxygen and sometimes, in the case of diabetics, sugar or juice administered orally.

For the EMT, the thought process is linear: Protect the patient at the scene; get her into the ambulance safely; then get to the hospital doing what you can as you go by providing simple, mechanical support to alleviate pain and prevent further injury and death.

Most of the physical care takes place inside the ambulance and is limited by the time it takes to get from the scene to the hospital. At times, during long-distance trips to the hospital, there's too much time! Without advanced care to offer, the EMT can only play witness to the inexorable march of death.

The paramedic, however, uses a circular process that involves observation, analysis, priority-setting, organization, communication, reception, modification, action and then back to observation. The cycle repeats itself until the patient is released to the care of the hospital.

Paramedics are responsible for all the functions of an EMT. Ultimately, they are responsible for the patient which means they're responsible for the *actions* of their EMT partners as well.

While regularly focusing on the patient and managing all of the things an EMT must, the paramedic also pays attention to the heart monitor, IV site, IV drip chamber, oxygen level, the drug box, and the radio. The paramedic's hands work constantly. If they are not busy intubating, starting the IV, administering other medications or applying the M.A.S.T. suit for example, they are manipulating dials and gauges, taking vital signs, adjusting IV flow rates, setting up the next round of medications, and/or taking notes for the radio report.

Internally, the paramedic's thoughts run something like this:

- If "A" occurs, I need to be ready to administer drug A1.
- If "B" occurs, and then is followed by "A" again, I need to call in to the doctor, and then be ready to add on drug B2 and then be ready to go to A5.

- If "C" should happen after "B," then I better cut back on A5 and be ready to intervene with C6, and then I better check for "A" again so I can report to the doctor.

It is very easy to get lost in the technical world of advanced pre-hospital care. So easy, in fact, that often many of the crucial "basics" are momentarily forgotten.

There are things the EMT on a non-paramedic unit can learn within a few months that a new paramedic who moves from school directly into the back of a Mobile Intensive Care Unit may take years to figure out. In large part it has to do with being a healer.

When everything has been done, after the EMT's bag of tricks has been exhausted — and that happens very quickly — all that's left is to be with the patient. Often, out of sheer frustration at having nothing left to do, the EMT discovers where the true power of healing lives.

For the paramedic, for whom it is easy to hide behind all the equipment and all the therapeutic choices that can be made, sometimes it takes a strong object lesson to act as a reminder of just how potent the role of an EMT can be.

"Lordy," Jerry said, "people sure don't know how to deal with wet 'round here, do they?"

It was a surprisingly calm statement, considering he just had to jerk the ambulance halfway into an intersection against the red light to avoid getting rear-ended by a skidding car.

As soon as I felt the lurch of the unit, heard the sliding car and its horn and the beginning of Jerry's comment, I quickly hit the emergency light switch — as if that would have made a difference. It's funny what rituals medics believe will protect them!

"Clear right," I said, as soon as I saw there was no cross traffic on my side. Still, had there been, I felt confident that Jerry would have been able to handle it. He was a damn good EMT.

I was partial to Jerry. He decided there was too much to learn. When he was offered a spot in the paramedic class after three months in the field as an EMT, he turned it down. "Give me a year," he said, "to see if I'm ready."

"You'd think by the third day," I commented, "people'd get used to rain." We continued through the empty intersection and headed toward Mission Santa Barbara.

"Not here," Jerry said, "it's much too…foreign." We were on our way Code 2 (urgent, non-emergency) for a tourist with a sprained ankle. That's good, I thought, I can let Jerry handle it if he wants. I'd let Jerry do anything he wanted. I trusted him to be self-limiting and set his own pace.

Moments in the Death of a Flesh Mechanic...a healer's rebirth

"Only vacationers would come out in lousy weather like this," I offered, "just to protect their investment."

"For sure," said Jerry, "look at it, 'cept for that idiot that almost rammed us, we're about the only car out on the road, and it's three o'clock in the afternoon. Damn near cripples commerce!"

That was amazingly true, I thought as I killed the emergency lights. It's as if the whole town hides when it rains. Everything takes on a pall that is so uncharacteristic of Santa Barbara. The streets look it — deprived of sun and covered with a veneer of mud-slime washing down the hills that's so very dirty for Santa Barbara! And being around the people you can feel it, kind of like bad weather means their birthright had been taken away from them.

Santa Barbara was not designed with rain in mind. Its streets provide the only real drainage for torrential rains coming down from the surrounding hillsides. The few sewage drains are woefully inadequate to the task. In heavy rains, water runs to and over curbs, flooding street corners and making the highway underpasses un-navigable by anything other than row boats! At the base of its many hills, torrents of water churn in vortex-like spirals as soon as they hit level ground.

Santa Barbara is synonymous with "light and airy". Its colors are bright and soothing. The dominant Spanish architecture — reddish clay tiled roofs draped over stucco walls — could be called "Sunny Weather Architecture." The people live between counting on exceptional weather and taking it for granted. You'd be hard pressed to find 50 umbrellas and raincoats in a thousand homes.

Rain disrupts everything about the normal rhythm of life in Santa Barbara. My thought was confirmed by dispatch. As soon as we pulled into the wide driveway leading to the imposing Spanish pueblo-style mission, our radio squawked.

"Medic Four, your 20?" A woman's voice came across the radio. It was Carol. She always sounded such a by-the-numbers pro that I could picture her barking terse instructions to her husband on their wedding night.

"Medic Four's 10-97 at the mission," Jerry replied.

"Reroute, Medic Four. Please proceed Code Three to a call for difficulty breathing at 2235 Mountain Drive. Repeat. Code Three, 2235 Mountain Drive. County Fire has been dispatched. Thomas Brothers 19, C, five. That's Charley, five. Confirm receipt of info Medic Four."

"Medic Four copys," Jerry replied.

I hit the lights and readied the siren as Jerry faded right, hopped the flooded curb in front of the Mission's fountain and pulled a U-turn.

Two men in trench coats came running out from the stucco and red tile-covered walkway leading to the church. They panicked at seeing us turn away. I would have yelled out something encouraging to them on the ambulance's

PA system, but I used it so rarely that I wasn't sure how to get it going without blasting them with the siren. I was embarrassed at our rudeness.

"They'll figure," Jerry said, reading my mind.

We sloshed out in front of the Mission and whipped left and crossed Foothill Road. Without any traffic to impede us, we made very good time.

We passed the county fire station, and proceeded just a short hop up the hill, and turned onto a gravel driveway that ended in a stand of eucalyptus trees about an eighth of a mile up the drive snaking across a field. Once we got past the trees, we saw two houses and a fire truck parked between them.

The larger of the houses was an uncompleted, three-story A-frame with a large porch and deck jutting out from the second level. Its beautiful redwood glistened in the rain. Redwood, now that's "Rainy Architecture," I thought.

To its rear was a weather-beaten, gray mottled, rectangular, two-story home. It, too, had a porch on its second level, supported by five rickety four-by-four beams. This house was literally on its last legs. Its upcoming fate was obvious.

A very well-dressed man jumped out from under the porch of the old home and, motioning us to follow him, he double-stepped the long set of stairs on the side of the house to its second level.

We called in 10-97 and grabbed our drug box, respiratory box, radio, Lifepak 5™, and oxygen and bounded up the stairs behind him.

At about the sixth rickety step, my right foot slid out from under me. I thrust the radio forward and to the side with my left arm to regain my balance. Luckily, it wedged between two widely spaced wooden slats of the guardrail and prevented me from falling backward. I was panting as I got to the second level.

The man who had led us in was standing in the living room, brushing the water off his perfectly pressed suit. It was clear that this was not his home because all the furniture was old and natty. He simply pointed to an open door, and then he sat down on a couch and cradled his head in his arms.

When he did that, my ears automatically perked up because I saw that he was covering his own. I immediately recognized the sounds of firemen nervously setting things up. One was calling out in panicked concern, "Just try and calm down, lady. It'll be all right."

Above the commotion, however, I heard a tortuous gurgling sound that pierced the room. I let Jerry enter the room first. I paused outside the door for a second to compose myself.

The sound I heard was the signature of someone drowning in her own bodily fluids; congestive heart failure. As distinctive a sound as there could be, at that intensity, it could only mean she was walking a tightrope over infinity.

In the room, Jerry had already opened the drug box and pulled out the blood pressure cuff. He was trying to make his way in-between two firemen who were standing on either side of a woman in her 60s. She was sitting on the very edge of a bed and holding on to the arms of an aluminum walker.

One of the firemen was trying to hold an oxygen mask on to the woman's face. He was doing his very best, it was obvious, but the situation was confusing to him. It was etched in every line of his face.

The woman was rocking back and forth on the edge of the bed. She was desperately caught. She was trying to stretch her chest up and forward so she could get more air into her lungs, and then, exhausted from the effort, she had to sit back and collapse. The see-saw motion was unnerving. When she had a semblance of balance, she batted the fireman's hand away from her face.

"Get...get that thing a...away from me." She gurgled and coughed. "I ca...can't br...breathe."

The fireman was looking at her imploringly.

"But, lady," he said, "it's oxygen. It'll *help* you breathe; please!" He tried to get the mask on her face. She bat his hand away again.

The fireman's partner, on the other side of the woman, didn't know whether to help her sit down or make her stand up. He stood alongside her with his arms outstretched, like a basketball player trying to limit the motions of his opponent without getting busted for a foul!

This was bad. There was much that needed to be done, and this woman was going to fight us every step of the way. No blame here. She was struggling for every breath. Where the hell was Jerry? I thought. He should have had me a line set up and the radio set up already. Wait a minute; I've got the damn radio.

Jerry came into view as he slowly stood up between the woman and the fireman. He was trying to position her. The look of concentration on his face was as intense as any I had ever seen. He was looking at her and taking in everything around her, too. He handed the fireman a blood pressure cuff and gently took the woman's arm and swung it out to him.

"Please," he said to the fireman.

Jerry took hold of the other fireman's hand. Carefully, he pulled it back about six inches away from her mouth and nose, and with it, the mask. Reaching across the fireman, he tweaked the valve of the portable oxygen unit to full flow. The air whooshed out to the woman.

Jerry leaned over and started whispering softly in her ear.

I was on my own. Everyone else was busy with the woman. I looked at the array of boxes and other equipment that was there for me to use. Now, I had to open up the boxes, set up my IV, lay out my first line of drugs, set the monitor up to transmit a rhythm strip to the hospital, get out my intubation equipment in case, and, oh yeah, get another IV bag out for a piggy-back.

In the beginning of my career as a paramedic, I had been quite distrustful of all the equipment. Even though I often felt like a kid at Christmas, with all these toys to play with under the tree, I still had a basic technophobia, or, at least, a definite wariness.

That was the result of my very first ambulance call where I had full responsibility for a patient.

It was back in Queens, New York, in 1974. I had just finished my Advanced First Aid course from the Red Cross and was volunteering at the Flushing Community Volunteer Ambulance Corps.

My brief internship with one of the more experienced medics was over, and, as usual, I was hanging out at the station hoping there would be a call. The primary ambulance was on a car wreck, and the attendant for the backup unit had just called in, unable to do his shift.

To my joy, another call came in, and it was my turn to act as the "patient man." The assignment was to transfer a patient from a local hospital to one in Manhattan, 15 miles away.

At the hospital in Flushing, I found my patient was a man in his late 70s who was just about comatose. The staff on duty, as often happens, just wanted him out so they could fill the bed with one of the three patients waiting to get in. The nurse in charge, not taking us seriously — none really did back then — just handed me his chart and helped us move him over to our gurney.

In the ambulance, a beautifully converted Cadillac hearse that still had that new car smell, the driver, Max, helped me get ready. I wrapped a BP cuff around the man's arm and pumped it up a little to help me hear the pulsations. The sounds I heard were weak.

I mentioned to my partner I was afraid I'd have a hard time monitoring the patient in the moving ambulance. He reached into one of the side compartments and pulled out what looked like a thick black plastic, hinged clothespin with elongated jaws. He handed it to me.

"Here," Max said, "Use this. It's a pulse monitor."

I turned it over in my hands, in awe at holding my first piece of high-tech equipment.

"It's brand new," he said. "We're doing evaluations of it for the manufacturer. It's a formality; damn thing works like a charm!"

Max showed me how to put it on the index finger of the man's left hand. As soon as it was on, a little red light on its surface started to blink on and off. I was fascinated.

Moments in the Death of a Flesh Mechanic...a healer's rebirth

"That's his pulse," Max told me, "a sensor picks up the..., um, pulsations I guess."

Still, before we moved, I pumped up the cuff again and listened to the man's faint heartbeat just to check. Sure enough, the monitor light and the heartbeat were in perfect harmony. So off we went.

Unfortunately, it was into a Friday night's rush hour traffic, and it was raining. This highway was one huge bottleneck. Max decided to use lights and siren all the way so that we'd make some sort of progress. A lot of good that did; this was New York City!

I just kept staring at those pulsations as the ambulance stopped and started, veered left and right, stopped and waited. Hadn't the nurse said "just make sure his heart doesn't stop?" Amazing, I thought; that monitor was catching every beat and I didn't have to worry about trying to find the pulse every few minutes! What will they come up with next?

Forty-five minutes later — to go fifteen miles, with lights blazing and siren blasting! — we pulled up to the hospital. My partner opened the back door, took one look at the patient and said, "I better go get someone," and ran off.

Taking a better look at the patient myself, I wondered if he wasn't looking kind of bad; like a whole lot worse than when we put him in. Was that blue around his lips? Wait a minute; now that the ambulance wasn't bouncing around, it didn't look like he was breathing! I went directly for his pulse at the carotid artery — as I had been trained to do with cardiac arrest — and there was none.

But the light was still flashing; slower than before, even steadier than before and with no uneven pauses. Confused, but knowing what I had to do, I snapped the head of the gurney down and gave him two mouth-to-mouth breaths without even looking for the Ambu-bag, and began chest compressions according to protocol. In the process, I knocked the little monitor off his finger, on to the floor. The light stopped blinking.

Within a very short period, Max was back with a doctor.

"Well," the doctor said, "we had high hopes that he'd get the boost he needed from the pacemaker. That wasn't the case — the muscle must've been gone, too. May as well stop, he's dead."

"Pacemaker?" I asked. My head was swimming with the little bit of information I just received.

"Yes," the doctor said.

He got into the back of the ambulance beside me and opened the man's pajama top. Just below the patient's left collarbone was a half-cigarette pack sized lump buried under the skin. It still had some fairly fresh sutures over it.

"They're still kind of new," the doctor said, "When the heart slows down to a dangerous level because it's missing too many beats; this pacemaker sends in a small electrical charge that stimulates the heart and causes it to beat when there's too long of a pause. It's probably still going. This guy would have been dead months ago if it weren't for this."

I just sat and stared. The doctor got out of the ambulance and he and Max went to get the morgue table. I fished under the gurney for the pulse monitor. I put it around the man's finger. The little bastard started flashing like a charm! It worked off of electrical activity; but in this case, it was one machine responding to another.

Perhaps this was why, even to that day, I always relied on my tactile senses first, used the machines I had available to me and then double-checked with my senses to be sure. At this house, even though most of my peers were automatically putting on gloves at the scene in response to the growing AIDS crisis, I did not take the time to do so.

I wedged the phone between my shoulder and head and then attached a line to an IV bag while I spoke to St. Francis Hospital.

"Doctor Sloan, we're on the scene with an approximately 65-year-old woman in acute respiratory distress. I'll need to be talked through this one on therapies. Please stand by."

I put the phone down and laid the IV bag and tubing on the drug box. I pushed the monitor, drug box and radio over toward the woman with my foot. The fireman called out her blood pressure. I handed him the cardiac monitor. I prayed he knew how to hook it up. Putting my stethoscope in my ears, I gently unbuttoned the back of the woman's dress and listened to her lungs.

The woman was still in a see-sawing motion. I could hear Jerry's soothing words, "Just concentrate on this breath. Don't worry about the next. Good; Now this one...Good!" I could hear her breathing relax. I shifted my attention from her lungs to her heartbeat. It was rapid.

Balancing the radio receiver again, I spoke to the doctor as I pulled the blood pressure cuff off and replaced it with a tourniquet.

"Status of the woman," I began. "In acute distress. Respirations are 24, very labored and irregular. Audible gurgling. Blood pressure 190 over 110. Pulse 80, irregular. Bilateral rales; crackling sounds more obvious left lung. Ankles swollen, severe on right. Cardiac rhythm..."

The monitor showed a wildly undulating line. The woman was surprisingly still. Jerry was still whispering to her. I checked her chest, which had been exposed, and saw one of the monitor patches had come loose. I pressed it on her, and it stuck long enough to show a regular beat followed by a PVC and then a flat line that was about twice the width of a normal beat.

"...ventricular bigeminii," I continued; "you want a strip?"

"Negative on that, Medic Four", the doctor replied. "Get the IV in. Admin 20 c.c.s Lasix, IV push. Follow with piggy-back aminophyllin, start with about 60 drops a minute. Get her here. En route, get a Lidoocaine bolus ready. Prepare a Lidocaine drip."

"I copy," I confirmed, "IV D5W TKO, Lasix, 20 c.c., Aminophyllin 500, piggy-back, 60 dpm and transport, continue to monitor with possibility of Lidociane drip. Our ETA is 15 minutes. Thank you, Dr. Sloan."

"Okay, see you soon." the doctor answered. The line went dead.

By now, things had calmed down just enough so that the woman had stopped rocking and shaking. I asked the firemen to find us a sturdy chair to get her down the stairs. Jerry let go of the woman's hand, which he was holding, and took the oxygen mask from the fireman. He asked me if I needed him to set me up as he put the mask fully on her face. She accepted it.

"Nuh-uh," I replied, "just do what you're doing."

And that he did. Jerry leaned close in to her, maintaining his chest even with hers. He calmly described everything I was going to do before I did it. The woman kept her eyes fixed straight ahead and was concentrating on every word that came out of his mouth. His complete and total attention was on her. By now, she had fallen into a regular breathing pattern; still noisy as hell, but steady. I noticed Jerry was maintaining equality with her. With his head parallel to hers, it looked like their faces were almost mirror images of each other. When she moved, he moved. It was almost like, yes, they were in synch. Jerry's calm was now being reflected by her.

That freed me to go back to the medical picture. Because of probable heart damage, the woman was not able to completely pump all the blood out of its left ventricle. Blood and fluid was now backing up into her lungs and suffocating her. The Lasix, a diuretic, would push her body to eliminate fluid. The aminophyllin would specifically target the backup in her lungs and help to strengthen her heart contractions.

It took me two attempts to get the IV started. After first I tried her hand and then blew a vein, Jerry said something to her. She looked at me and gave me a half-hearted, shaming snarl. Jerry chuckled. I didn't take a chance on a second attempt on her hand, and went right for the antecubital region of her arm; inside the bend of her elbow, an area you usually save after all other secondary veins have been used or blown.

The needle seated properly, and after carefully anchoring the line and tubing, I broke open the two vials of Lasix, drew them up in a syringe and injected them into the IV tubing. While I was injecting the aminophyllin into its bag of fluid, the firemen came with a chair.

Before the aminophyllin was piggy-backed to the IV, she was sweating profusely; the Lasix had kicked in. Jerry, taking the cue, asked if we could move her over into an old, wooden straight-backed chair the firemen had brought.

"Be care...careful," she said, barely audibly, "tha...that's the last...one of my moth...mother's dining room set."

She smiled, seeming to be happy to have been able to get anything out at all. Jerry draped his arms around her reassuringly. She shifted to the chair. Although in distress, she was much more secure now.

The aminophyllin started kicking in, too, I thought.

Jerry took off his raincoat and draped it over her. She looked at him and shook her head "No." He squeezed her arm. "Yes," he said

Jerry and the firemen brought her out of the house and down the stairs to the stretcher that the Firemen had set up at the foot of the steps. I accompanied them on the way down, worrying over the monitor. Because of the movement, I couldn't be sure if the erratic blips on the screen were from the motion or due to a potentially fatal aberration.

The monitor; check the woman's consciousness; the monitor; the IV; the oxygen. The This, the That, the Other...while Jerry was doing nothing more than being with her completely, and that's what was getting her down the stairs!

When I was sure everything was stable enough, I ran back up the stairs to grab my equipment. Her son was waiting for me.

"I don't want you to think I don't care," he apologized, "she's... things, things were so...so scary, I couldn't watch."

I picked up my suction equipment and airway box. I handed him the drug box.

"Yes," I replied, "it was pretty scary. You weren't wrong. But it's a lot better now." I led him onto the porch in the rain. He followed me down the stairs.

"See," he said, "that's why I'm building the new house. At least I can be close by. I can do that. Get her a nurse, which I can do." He was trying to convince me.

All I could think to do was to look him in the eyes and smile. So I did.

"You know, you saved her life," he concluded

Before I could control it, at the base of the steps, the word "bullshit" came out of my mouth. Not angrily or loud, just a matter-of-fact comment. It just came out. It startled both of us.

"All I did," I countered quickly and in as friendly a way as I could so as not to insult him, "was play mechanic."

I tossed my load of equipment into the back of the ambulance, and then, grabbing the drug box from his hands, I placed it inside the unit and opened it so I could pull drugs out if I needed them. I did a mental check to be sure I hadn't forgotten anything. I hadn't.

Moments in the Death of a Flesh Mechanic...a healer's rebirth

After helping the man into the passenger seat of the ambulance, I went to the side door. Jerry was sitting on the jump seat by the patient, working with her. They were calmly breathing in unison.

I was the paramedic. I was the one who had to ride in the back with the patient. All I did was plug in a few tubes and squirt a couple drugs into them. I had nothing to do with the patient. And now, I had to trade places with Jerry, and he was what was keeping her alive.

Without any resistance to leaving because he knew he was the driver, Jerry leaned over to the woman and said, "Russ is going to ride in with you." He looked at me and nodded. "And he's going to do what I've been doing."

I got partially in to the back and took the oxygen mask from him and, like I saw Jerry was doing, held it about an inch from her mouth and nose. He slipped behind me and out of the back, closing the door behind him. I, of course double-checked the oxygen level, the IV site and the flow rates. The ambulance started moving. I saw I had nothing left to do. I leaned over to the woman.

"Um..." I stammered, "how're ya doin'?"

I had no idea where my hand was until she gently pushed it and the mask off of her face so she would have room to answer.

"Fine...better." She said and then clamped her hand around mine and held it steady, with the mask about one inch from her face as Jerry had done. And then she just took slow and easy breaths as she kept her eyes fixed on the rear door of the unit.

She'd do fine, as long as I could follow in Jerry's footsteps. I realized for the first time in a long time, I was jealous of my partner.

Chapter Twelve
TUG OF WAR

"Cuyama?" I asked, "I've heard of New Cuyama in the sticks. There's an old one besides?"

"There is a Cuyama," Don replied. "About two miles the other side of New Cuyama."

"I expect there's a tremendous difference between the two."

"Sure, Cuyama's got the gas station!"

We were on our way 60 miles inland to do a routine transfer of a cardiac patient for admission to a hospital in Santa Maria. I was happy to have the call. It gave me a chance to visit another part of this oddly diverse county.

The particular area we were going to was out in the middle of an extremely arid strip of land nestled in between a couple of mountain ranges; a tremendous contrast to lush Santa Barbara to the southwest and the highly cultivated farmlands around Santa Maria to the west

The Cuyamas had a reputation. High-speed wrecks were their signature calls. Some lonely traveler would be scooting along Highway 33 at four o'clock in the morning when he'd see what looked like fresh tire tracks leaving the tarmac and ripping through the sand into a patch of shrubbery, a ditch, or even the rare tree. The poor traveler would zip by, then, shaking the sleep from his eyes, ask himself, "Did I see that?"

He'd go back to check. Sure enough, there'd be the remnants of a car, upside down, almost unrecognizable; the aftermath of something that happened hours ago. The people were mincemeat. The traveler would be hard-pressed to find a telephone, and unless someone could be left at the scene who knew how to stabilize, the time delay would often be fatal.

Once notified, both the Cuyama based County Fire Department ambulance (EMT) and a paramedic unit in Santa Maria was dispatched. The Fire medics would begin stabilization and then load the patients up and head balls to the wall for Santa Maria, sixty or so miles away.

Moments in the Death of a Flesh Mechanic...a healer's rebirth

The two units would usually meet at about the halfway point on Highway 166, some 30 or so miles out of Santa Maria. Then, the patients would be transferred to the paramedic unit and stabilized as best as could be (or stabilized in the Fire unit before transferring to the paramedic rig), and then the last leg of the transfer would begin.

There was an average of one medical or trauma related call per month in the Cuyama Valley. That was a problem. With three shifts in the fire department, the odds were high that each Fire EMT would be exposed to only one medical call every three months; a volume too low to allow one to keep up his emergency skills. By the time the paramedic unit would meet the fire department rig, more often than not, the patients would be going sour and the EMT's would be scared half to death.

Considering all the horror stories I had heard, this little routine transfer was a pleasure. But, naturally, there is a divine sense of humor at work in everything, and we were rolling right into the heart of it!

Space; so much space and brown/gray dryness with just enough moisture in the soil to prevent it from being cracked and parched, but not enough to support anything green. I lifted my feet and stretched them out on to the cowling of the Ford Econoline's engine. Leaning back in my seat, I just let the ride take me; time passing as a ribbon of miles.

The radio broke in on my serenity.

"Medic Eight," the dispatcher said, "new information."

"Go for Medic Eight." Don had picked up the mic.

"Your patient has gone," she continued, "by car to the hospital."

"We're about 15 minutes out," Don stated; "please advise."

"No fair," I said to Don, "I wanted to check out this place."

I wondered if it would take much to talk him into stretching the last few miles into town. No problem, I figured; Don's cool.

"Medic Eight," the dispatcher came back, "I guess, proceed until I can confirm — there seems to be some confusion here."

"Ten-four," Don replied.

Almost immediately, the dispatcher came back with, "Medic Eight, step it up to Code Three. Apparently the family drove the patient to the fire station. It sounds like a Code Blue. Your ETA?"

"Eight minutes," Don answered immediately. "and 42 seconds."

In no time we were going a hundred miles an hour and my casual tour had become a high-speed careen through the valley. Pulling out of a curve from sandy gray-brown, open fields at the base of a mountain, suddenly we came across a series of perfectly delineated, bright green circles of vegetation placed every half mile. Framed by the mountains on either side, each patch was the size of a football field.

Whoosh, a patch. Whoosh, barren soil. Whoosh, a patch.

My eyes darted back and forth from the road to the patches, trying to make sense of them and still be a good shotgun for my driver. Extending from a center post in each green circle was a thin plastic irrigation tube supported by tall, thin metal wheels every 10 yards or so, such that it could be rolled around the radius of its circle.

It all seemed so organized and logical, clearly the work of man

After five minutes of tense driving, dispatch chimed in again

"Medic Eight," she said, "cut back to Code Two. County fire reports the patient is fine. Proceed to the station."

We were almost there, so we kept on into the more populated area with our lights on, but no siren. More populated means one house every quarter mile, a barn, a garage, and a bare lot holding farm machinery. The dominant gray flowed into a patch of fenced in, sickly green and brown mottled pastures. In the distance were black blotches scattered about that seemed oddly unlike cows

"What the fuck'er them?" I asked my partner.

"Buffalo."

"Right," I replied.

He didn't have to respond. We passed a restaurant where one had no place being. Advertised on its white fence a sign blared out, "BUFFALO STEAKS, BUFFALO BURGERS, BUFFALO FRIES!"

Sure enough, I could see in the pasture that they were buffalo, right in the middle of Santa Barbara County when, at the time, they barely could be found in the prairies of South Dakota!

"Nice joke," I said. "I thought they were endangered."

"Obviously!" Don shrieked at me.

Now I was confused, but it didn't matter. Just as we got within a block of the dusty little fire station, dispatch called us again.

"Medic Eight, your patient's in cardiac arrest... ETA?"

"We're there." I pulled the mic this time while Don maneuvered the rig into the driveway, close by the open bay doors.

I jumped into the back of the ambulance and started tossing equipment onto the gurney. Don pulled the gurney out, and we both rolled it through the garage to a door that leads to the reception area.

Moments in the Death of a Flesh Mechanic...a healer's rebirth

Most medics get trained by experience to size up the atmosphere of a room in the time it takes to get their face through the door. It is instant hyperawareness where a sort of radar gets turned on. The radar takes in what can't be seen but only felt.

It's the same skill that a kid picks up when she lives in a dysfunctional home. If dad's drunk, she notes where he is in the house, where the closest exit is, his emotional state and especially if he's primed to strike. She must, because her survival depends on it. She is attuned.

Pacing is important, especially in how you enter the room. In a room full of panicky people, you enter swiftly and surely, in control. In a room with the distraught, move with the flow of what's there. Blend in and find your place, but with strength. In one filled with anger, you make sure you enter smoothly, rock solid and without hesitation.

Once in the room, move to the center of the scene without disrupting the balance present. Most often, there is plenty of chaos. In that case, you become the hub of the wheel and set the "tone" of the scene. The important thing is to move like you have everything under control. It's a matter of managing the elements so you have to deal with as few variables as possible while you get your patient stabilized and out.

So much of that success is dependent on the way you and your partner interrelate. Each of you is, essentially, working the room. The degree to which you can establish a zone of security, safety and control in the space between you will determine how smoothly the call goes.

This is an art that takes years to develop for most. Some medics are naturals; some stay relatively oblivious of their surroundings for a painfully long time. In either case, there are many subtleties to master.

Take, for example, working with other vital protection agencies, like police and firemen. You don't just barrel into a scene as if you're boss. Even knowing things are chaos, a cooperative, even ingratiating stance is the order of the day. Good politics dictates that.

Don and I paused at the doorway the briefest moment to assess the scene. Three firemen were on their knees on the floor. An oxygen cylinder was stretched out alongside a swarthy man in coveralls, lying on his back. He looked about 70. The man's coverall top had been pulled down, shirt ripped open, and what looked to be a fresh bruise right in the center of his chest, over his sternum.

What was confusing, however, was all the firemen seemed to be elated. They were looking at each other with congratulatory smiles, and then back to the man, who seemed to be holding court.

"Granddaughter's weddin'," he said, "what that run us, Emmie?"

He questioned a woman who was clearly a rancher's wife. She was wearing an old topcoat touching all the way to the floor. Looking up to the ceiling in thought, she didn't seem at all upset.

"Oh," she said, "I'd say about two...no...Twenty-five hundred."

What the hell was going on? I asked myself. Had we walked into a bizarre coffee klatch? I couldn't find where I belonged.

"Yup...." said the man, "I'd say that's about it..." He looked up and noticed us. "Well, hello boys," he said, "what's the hubbub?"

A fireman got up and motioned Don and me out to the garage.

"He's 72," said the fireman whose name tag introduced him as Ben. "He's had occasional chest pain on exertion for the last two months. They did testing at Marian and wanted him to come in for a bypass. Nothing had gotten to where he was in danger, I guess. The trip was uncomfortable for him last time. He didn't like his wife's driving, so they scheduled you guys to transport. His name is Roy McArthur."

The fireman had a shit-eating grin on his face. He was proud of something. It was infectious, and I found myself grinning back at him.

"Anyway," Ben continued, "about a half-hour ago, he started to have chest pain. His wife decided to get him into the car and over to here. As she opened the door for him, he collapsed and hit the floor, flat on his back. She yelled out to him, but he didn't answer. Panicking, she punched him as hard as she could, right in the chest."

"Just like on TV!" Don interjected as he went back into the room, "I'll hook him up to the monitor. Get the rest of the report, Russ."

"Yeah," Ben said, "like on the old shows. So the odd part is he just snapped out of it! I wonder if he just didn't fall and she freaked out. She helped him back into the car and brought him here."

"Someone from the house must have called it in," I said. "We got stepped up to Code Three."

"She came in," Ben went on, "and, while he sat in the car, she told us all this. Just when she's talking about him snapping out of it, he comes walking in the door bitching about hospital and ambulance bills, then, out of nowhere, he falls out in front of me. Boom: Hits the floor!"

Ben pointed down to his feet, as if the man were still there.

"I jumped right on him," he said, "No breathing. NO pulse. I extended his neck, gave him a couple of breaths and then started compressions. I got to about the fifth compression..."

"And he snapped out of it?" I asked.

Moments in the Death of a Flesh Mechanic...a healer's rebirth

"You betcha," Ben went on proudly, "not only that, he picked up his conversation right where he left off. That's where you came in."

"Far out," was all I could think to say.

My sixth sense told me to do the strategizing away from the patient. Besides, all was under control, jocular even. I wondered if his wife and the fireman both misinterpreted what was going on with him. Poor bastard got beat around a bit. Still, he seemed no worse for wear.

I went and got the radio and brought it into the garage. I called the hospital while Don brought me the rhythm strip he had run on the patient. He gave me an update on vital signs, which were good.

The strip showed quite a few PVCs — premature ventricular contractions. Many of them perilously close to the recharging phase.

The way it works is the heart beats because an electric stimulus comes in and starts a wave of contractions in its cells. Just like when you give your arm an electrical shock, the muscle cells contract and you twitch. After each beat, the heart goes through a resting phase to prepare for the next contraction. While the heart muscle is recharging, if another electrical stimulus comes in too early, it begins a wave of contractions that run counter to the last wave. Each cell begins beating independently, out of synch with the others as if 100 people in a 20' X 20' room all started for *different* exit doors at once! This causes fibrillation; the heart quivers rather than pumps, thereby stopping effective blood flow.

There definitely is something cooking here, I thought, though I still had a hard time believing the man had just gone into cardiac arrest. I relayed the information to the doctor and received orders for an IV and a 10 cc bolus (pre-loaded IV injection) of Lidocaine — a drug that reduces the irritability of the heart. He also ordered a piggy-back of Lidocaine; a slower infusion to assure the patient gets a steady dose of the drug. Today, this approach is out of favor.

There was certainly enough help. The patient was so calm and gay even, that Don was able to get the therapies going without a problem.

One of the fireman asked if we could replace their nasal oxygen cannulas with some from our stock. Don also saw the monitor batteries were getting very low, so he pulled them and went to get replacements. The firemen and I positioned the gurney near the man.

On his way out, Don brought the patient's wife into another room; a truly inspired move. No sooner had they left and we had begun to lift the patient, when, sure enough, the man's eyes rolled back and skyward and saying, "Huh?" he went limp.

Without hesitating, I let the body slide out of my arms back onto the floor, grabbing to support his head so it wouldn't bounce.

"Mug him," I called out to Ben.

One of the most enjoyable things about becoming a paramedic at the time was you could delegate. The first thing you did was to have others do mouth-to-mouth for you if the situation demanded it.

Up to the mid-80s, it wasn't uncommon to do mouth-to-mouth resuscitation, in the field, without protection. If you didn't have an Ambu-bag, which has a mask on it, then you wrapped your mouth around the patients' and began breathing for them. Protection wasn't a necessity as it is today. With the advent of new CPR techniques, even breathing for the patient is not as critical a component as it once was!

There were many devices designed to act as barriers between you and the patient or as an adjunct to maintaining an open airway. Still, many of us in the field then couldn't be bothered using them. They were complex to assemble and prone to come apart at the worst of times, often causing an obstruction which is what they were designed to prevent!

An example was the Esophageal Obturator Airway (EOA). You'd insert a hollow plastic tube into the patient's esophagus. The tube had a plug on its far end and holes near its top. You'd inflate a "cuff" around the tube, anchoring it in the esophagus. You put more air in the cuff than with the endotracheal tube because the cuff had to expand to occupy the wider passage of the esophagus. The benefit was you didn't have to visualize the vocal cords. Basically, you were pushing in a plug so nothing could come up from the stomach and get in to the lungs.

Then, you'd attach a mask to the tube and strap it to the patient's head (with rubber straps that often ripped!) and push in air with a bag mask. With nowhere else to go, the air would go into the patient's lungs. The problem was, at the end of the call, often you'd find the tube had separated from the mask and pushed deep into the patient's stomach!

Nothing was less glamorous than wrapping your mouth around some stranger's ("mugging") and getting the blowback of matter from his lungs or stomach into your own mouth. Yet, assembling or positioning a device while the patient was apneic looked far worse!

Ben didn't question me. He sprung right into action. Often, you'd get this "Oh, shit! Do I hafta?" look. He could have just jumped on doing compressions, an old trick, and motioned a less experienced fireman to do the mugging, but he chose not to.

I had my endotracheal tube and laryngoscope ready by the time Ben finished his third breath into the patient. In the meantime, Don, caught off guard, fumbled and almost dropped all the things he was carrying — a short wooden backboard to place on the gurney under the man's back to support CPR, the nasal cannulas and the batteries.

I took my place to control the airway. Ben went to chest compressions calling out "One and two and three and four and..." with each one as he did so. The monitor image was all over the place. I saw one of the electrodes flopping around, unattached to the patient.

I got ready to ask Ben to stop for about 30 seconds so I could insert the endotrachael tube, and then I thought I saw the man move his hand. I looked to Ben to see if perhaps he was being too rough in his compressions. He was not. This is what I heard:

Ben — "Eight and nine and..."

Patient — "What th..."

Ben — "Ten and..."

Patient — "Hell..."

Ben — "E-le..."

Patient — "are you..."

Ben — "Jesus Christ... Mr. McArthur...I'm sorry!"

Before Don even had a chance to charge up the defibrillator paddles, the patient had awakened. Ben was looking down at him in terror; his hands pulled back at shoulder level as if to say, "These? No, these weren't the hands crushing your chest, sir!"

Don reattached the electrodes. We saw the rhythm strip was unchanged — even after the meds had been put on board. The drugs should have kicked in by now. This call was getting interesting.

"Mr. McArthur," I said evenly, "we're going to be moving things quick here for a minute. Bear with us and everything'll be fine."

He looked up at me, confused. I was glad…just enough so a little reassurance would go a long way and he'd cooperate.

"Into to the rig, boys," I called out, "Now!"

Don elevated the head of the gurney while I placed my arms under the patient's armpits and took his left wrist in my right and right in my left hands, and crossing his arms, lifted him up while the firemen supported his legs. Mr. McArthur was on the gurney and wheeled out. It was customary, on long calls like this, to have one of the firemen assist on the trip. Ben got into the back with me.

"You're up for this, "I asked.

"Absolutely," was his reply.

As we got organized and the ambulance started moving, I saw Mrs. McArthur, sitting in front, craning her neck in to look back at her husband. Apparently satisfied, she pulled her head back, and as soon as she did, Don closed the compartment door that separates the cab from the rear of the ambulance.

I called in to the hospital. The doctor ordered continuous monitoring and EKG transmission to the hospital. Mr. McArthur, less talkative, was still bright-eyed. As we were sending the signal, he was looking around the ambulance as if trying to get his bearings. I noticed a slowing of his heart rate followed by a PVC, then a pause, then a beat and before the beat was finished. Bam! a PVC landed smack on the first third of the "T" wave, the recharging phase.

Mr. McArthur went, "Unh," and unconscious. This time, the positive pressure breathing mask was ready. Ben snapped the head of the stretcher down and began ventilating the man. I was charging the paddles when the doctor came in over the radio.

"I saw." he said. "Don't hit him with 360 joules. Start at 50."

With the older Lifepak™ models, once the charge button is pushed, you can't cancel it until the full charge is reached. You have to wait until they're charged, then discharge, then charge again at the new setting. I had to go through the process. Each second felt like an hour.

As soon as Ben gave his three respirations, he saw I wasn't ready and went right into compressions again. He was going about it a lot more attentively now. His eyes were riveted on the man's face.

At his sixth compression, I was ready. I had Ben move away, placed the paddles on Mr. McArthur's chest and discharged them. Unlike a discharge at full capacity, the 50 joules were not enough to cause the patient's muscles to contract, thereby making the body hop on the gurney. Instead, there was only a little "pop!" with no movement following.

We waited to see what was showing on the screen. There was no return to normal rhythm. Ben ventilated the man once more and then began compressions again while I spoke to the doctor.

"Let's go to 75," he said. "I want to find this guy's threshold. Run the piggyback full flow, charge and then defibrillate."

As the paddles charged, I heard Mr. McArthur calling out, "No...Oh!...please..." in rhythm with Ben's compressions. There seemed to be a time lag between the time the patient regained consciousness and the time the message got through to Ben's hands to stop compressing.

Now, Mr. McArthur reached up to push Ben's hands away from his chest. Poor Ben was as pale as a ghost.

"Good job. Medic Eight," said the doctor; "he's converted."

Movement of the ambulance combined with interference from compressions must have wiggled the monitor line enough to obscure the signal — enough so that he thought we had defibrillated again.

"That was CPR, doc," I said, "didn't have a chance to defib."

" Next time he goes," Dr. Gilroy replied. "be ready with 75."

Moments in the Death of a Flesh Mechanic...a healer's rebirth

"Hit him with 75. Ten-four," I repeated,

"No," Mr. McArthur called out, "*Don't* hit me anymore!"

"Um, Mr. McArthur," Ben stumbled with his words unconvincingly, "that was something else they were talking about."

Apparently tiring, the patient did not respond.

"Better cut back the Lidocaine," the doctor called in.

Shit. I almost forgot. There were fewer PVCs on the monitor now, but every time one showed up, it was sure close to that "T" wave. Nothing to do except sit, and watch, and wait.

Sure enough, within five minutes, as we passed those green crop circles, another PVC landed on the hot spot, and Mr. McArthur passed out. This time, I charged up and defibrillated immediately, even before Ben could begin compressions. I was fascinated by seeing the rogue beat hitting the "T" wave right on that vulnerable spot. I was always part of the aftermath. Did I mention how much I loved stuff like that?

No luck. Ben gave respirations and started CPR while the doctor said, "Go for a hundred," which I did. No luck.

Ben's compressions were not forceful now; he was hesitating. While I administered another bolus of Lidocaine, I told him to deepen his compressions. He did, with a look of renewed determination on his face. His third compression produced a loud CRAAACK!

"Oh, God!" Ben exclaimed.

"Keep going," I barked. "It's just a rib."

No one tells you in your CPR class what it's going to feel like when ribs start cracking under your hands. There are few words to describe it because the crack occurs underneath living flesh. It's bound to happen. With the aged, it's almost a given. No matter how perfectly you are positioned, no matter how careful, and no matter the age of the patient, if you do CPR enough, it will happen. Some medics say if you're not breaking ribs, you're not doing it right.

Ben kept on. I placed the paddles and readied to discharge 150 joules. Mr. McArthur came back. He groaned out, "Ohhh...Owww!"

Ben had been leaning over the patient doing his compressions. He let himself fall back into a sitting position on the squad bench. Mr. McArthur laid back and seemed to fall asleep. "What the hell is going on here?" Ben asked.

"Dunno," I said. "No response to Lidocaine or cardioversion. Appears to be on a whacky timetable; maybe next round we can..."

"I don't care about that," Ben interrupted. "Why in the hell is this happening to ME?"

Uh-oh, I thought, he's taking this personally.

"It's actually happening to him," I whispered, trying to lighten the mood, deflect him a little. Ben would have none of it.

"It's like playing tug of war with God," he said, nodding toward Mr. McArthur, "*He's* just caught in the middle of the mess!"

Ben was angry. At first, I was startled. You usually don't make such statements amidst a call, but with this patient flip-flopping between being with us and being pulled away (pulled away? Did I think that? I guess I did.), what other conclusion could be drawn?

I had a sneaky suspicion if it were me on the delivering end of those compressions instead of Ben, things would be different; not that I would have done anything better. For some reason, this drama seemed slated to unfold with Ben being the focal point; as if God purposely put him and Mr. McArthur in an arena together. That was a chilling thought.

"Ben," I said as I took the blood pressure cuff off the patient's left arm and handed it to him, "I need a set of competing blood pressures; can you do that for me, please."

Ben got to work, but I could tell he wasn't quite sure what I had asked him to do. I counted on it. He fumbled with the cuff and stethoscope, taking readings from one arm and then the other, confused because he detected no difference. In that confusion, he stopped thinking.

"Lord...I feel so sore," Mr. McArthur said as he gingerly held his left side in pain and then opened his eyes.

"You just rest," Ben said to the man as he carefully worked around him; "everything will work out fine."

The major part of me was absolutely fascinated by the technical intricacies of what was going on. The patient was responding not at all the way he should have; no matter how much Lidocaine was put on board, the fatal beats kept coming. Not only that, but the patient didn't respond to electrical shock, only to manual compressions. Was it touch?

The man was snapping directly from clinical death into consciousness, back and forth, with what I could only call minimal disorientation and almost full presence. Each time he came back, the sparks in his eyes were present; not drifting away. What a show!

I knew that getting lost in the technical aspect helped me avoid getting pulled in to the emotional content of Ben's plight. Now *that* was genuine horror! The circumstances were so incredibly weird, though; it almost made sense that somebody experienced the emotion of what was happening. Unfortunately, Ben was at the center of the Bull's Eye.

This is common in emergency calls, and, indeed in small group dynamics. One person will *act out* the intense energy that is being *held in* by the others in the room. Sometimes grief, others fear or horror, anger or the like. Management of the scene includes identifying and dulling the impact of magnified emotion on the person susceptible to acting it out.

Everything happening must have been gruesome to Ben. The one in the most turmoil was the caregiver rather than the patient. I knew I was holding up the Flesh Mechanic end, and Ben, the human being side. They both had to be part of the game. The Mechanic's role was to channel Ben's emotional content without killing it. It was powering some precise work that no one in the world was in a better position to provide.

Personally I felt unaffected. Was it because many times I had traveled the territory where the dead pass on and leave the living to agonize? Perhaps. But more important, I sensed this was *Ben's* moment.

I had many of my own where I'd been forced to find a guiding philosophy to hold on to. It was either that or quit, and believe me, many have done so over just such dilemmas.

One day, I misdiagnosed a patient. I had been a paramedic for a month. I found him vomiting in a hotel room, wrapped around a toilet. His wife, who staggered to the door to meet me and my partner, said they had dinner and only a "couple" of drinks. Her husband had come back and gotten sick. He wasn't on meds and had no history of problems.

In his 50s, the man's body was loose. He was slurring words. He looked drunk. I wrote him off as drunk. His pulse was thready. He was sweating profusely, and I had a hard time getting a BP on him. All of these signs, to me, were consistent with someone in the throes of a solid pukefest. Even though I have a weak sense of smell, I detected an alcohol odor hovering in the toilet bowl. Was this not how I, myself, had been after a night that concluded with worshipping the porcelain God?

It was an inarguable decision, however, to bring him to the emergency room for a check. He fell silent, but was looking about as we carried him out on the stretcher. About halfway down the third flight of stairs, I looked up at him and began to think I had made a mistake; his color had suddenly turned ashen, though he was still breathing.

In the back of the ambulance, I decided to use some of the new paramedic equipment that I had been given. The call had come as a "visitor with stomach problems", so I hadn't lugged my heavy equipment up the stairs. I was still at the stage of using everything judiciously.

I hooked him up to the heart monitor to find the man was in what's called an "agonal" heart rhythm — the last throes of a heart that was ready to quit. He had been having a whopper of a heart attack when I first saw him and I had missed it!

Had I administered oxygen, contacted the hospital for orders, started an IV and administered the first round of drugs — atropine to speed up his heart — chances are he would have been stable enough to have tolerated the trip. As it was, the time he was left untreated combined with the stress of moving was pushing him over the edge.

Once I realized my mistake, I did spring into action. Then, a series of "accidents" began. I couldn't get through to the hospital. As my partner barreled through Daytona Beach on my Code Three request, I dropped protocol and just went for the IV without getting orders. In the rocking ambulance, I destroyed two of the three viable veins the man had in his body. I remember cursing God for setting me up. By the time I did get the line running, we had reached the hospital. I only administered oxygen and dextrose and water through the IV. It hardly mattered, by then the man was taking his last gasp.

There was nobody to meet us at the door of the emergency room, so we had to bring him in without help. We rolled him into the cardiac cubicle, and lo and behold, there were not one, but six doctors standing there! I thanked God for being around to bail me out.

Something came clear to me. If God had wanted this guy dead, He would not have had his wife call. We wouldn't have made the decision to transport. And since he had no history, he probably was weathering my minor mistakes. God had to have wanted this guy to live. Why else would there be six doctors there?

Boy was I wrong! As soon as the man was transferred on to the hospital gurney, he went into cardiac arrest.

First revelation; the doctors weren't doctors. They were interns; and green interns at that. I didn't realize this until I watched for a moment. It was sheer pandemonium. No one was in charge and no instructor came to bail them out. I doubted anybody knew what to do, but everyone sure wanted to get in there! It was obvious none of them had ever run a code on a real human before.

Not knowing how to handle the situation (these were kinda doctors weren't they? I couldn't just step in, could I?), I ended up slinking into the corner and watching what my incompetence reaped.

I talked to myself as if an announcer making exclamations at some sort of maudlin game where everything was going wrong: "Protect his airway! Turn his head to the side and sweep; he's still vomiting; Don't intubate while he still has shit coming out of his mouth! *Suction him, for God sakes!* Can't you see? Now, he's fibrillating. Defibrillate him. *Christ, not with 200 joules!* Go to a full 360. Oh, shit...the paddles go high right shoulder and low left side, not high left and low right!"

Frozen in my tracks, I watched as the interns threw away whatever chance the man had of surviving.

I agonized over that call for years. Why did God use me to kill him? I was the one with the responsibility. Why was I blinded? Why did everything I touch in the back of the rig turn to shit? Why, once I realized what was going on, did I feel kept away from doing anything to benefit the man in his final struggle? Why was I made to watch him die?

I had broken a sacred trust in a classic case of sudden death. This was what I was trained for as a paramedic. The man had a high probability of recovery, if he were caught in time. It was me, the rookie paramedic, the community's worst nightmare, who tossed his life away. I had failed, and because I failed, God was making me pay the price.

I could easily take this all personally. That would mean I was not worthy; that I blew it with him and I'd blow it again and was now a lightning rod for the twisted Gods! My quitting might actually *save* lives! The alternate was to find something to hang on to, a rationale that would help me to reconcile my role.

Somehow, I had to understand the Force I was working against. Having been an EMT with limited tools, I built up the mistaken belief that now, with all this great stuff to use, if the right mechanical things were done in the proper sequence at the right time, a life could be saved.

When everything is done right and the patient still dies, however, sometimes it does seem as if that life had been taken from you. It feels like the loss of a personal fight, even if you didn't have some personal investment in saving the life in the first place. In the back of your mind, you do wonder to yourself: Am I battling to keep on this earth something that God's calling back?

In the history of the world, for 99% of the people who've ever lived, when it was time to go, people just went. There was no one to intervene; no one properly trained to do the simplest thing, like clearing an airway to prevent choking. God's way mostly seems content with just letting life pass. It is the "sophisticated" cultures — the technologically advanced — who take it upon themselves to push the issue.

Still, cessation of life is inevitable; the way of God, Goddess, Mother Nature, Great Spirit, Higher Power — whatever you choose to call it. Maybe the way has nothing to do with by Whom; it just *is*.

At our very best, we can only delay death and that's a miracle! We're helping our patients to be part of an extremely select group. Only fractions of a fraction of a fraction of one percent of the people who have ever lived have ever had a chance of being "saved".

Because death is the way of all life, it cannot be personal. Who lives and who dies and when, where or how others participate is irrelevant; that's just the way it is.

So I determined that what I had gone through was not personal.

I was not sent to destroy the man. God did not have an in for him, or a hatred for me that put us together in such a painful way. God was not in a struggle against me — He, wanting the man alive and me, doing my best to kill him, and then, suddenly switching sides and Him taking the man for himself!

I was simply one of a number of things that sealed the man's fate. Timing was the only variable. Every thing that happened was a reflection of a greater reality — we all must die. The chilling thought was I purposely placed myself in the position where lives could easily slip through my hands if I missed or neglected something. But even that had to be a part of, "Nothing personal, kiddo; that's just the way it is!"

Yet, it was left to me to find a way to forgive myself in order to carry on. The only way I could conceive to do so was to make damn sure that such a mistake of negligence would never happen again.

Every subsequent call, for the rest of my career, had the presence of that man in it. It *was* a deeply personal experience. My life touched the last moments of his in a very profound way. And he, in turn, touched mine back. That particular life meant something to me. I wanted him to live. I mourned and felt loss — not only *of* him, but *in* me of a big layer of innocence. The incredible gift he gave me as his last act on earth was a full understanding of the stakes I was playing with.

He would not let me forget: Every time I was faced with a choice to get more meticulous or slack off, I chose the former as if he were standing by me, watching. It was nothing *but* personal, and never with a sense of threat. The man became, in some cases, my will to fight.

My relationship with that man in those moments left an indelible impression on me. His life force stayed with me. I credit him with being instrumental in my saving many more lives. Aboriginal cultures recognize the living influence of the spirits of their predecessors. Today, I understand better how that works.

The last moments of that man's life also prompted me to seek solace from a Power greater than myself. To my surprise, comfort was available to me when I asked for it. I stood at the feet of a very personal teacher who showed me that God's forgiveness means nothing in the here and now unless I made the effort to forgive myself. And the only way to make that happen was to take the lesson I learned and, rather than hide from it, to transform it into something useful for others.

So, now I find myself praying to what I know damn well is an impersonal God for the guidance She has for me personally.

Go figure.

This is why I had little to offer to Ben in his crisis. I simply kept his body going — busying his hands so his head would cease its disturbing chatter. I felt confident that he, too, would be guided to the right answer for him.

Ben was trying his best to choreograph his movements into a smooth flow. Still, I could sense the dread building up in him. He kept looking nervously back and forth from monitor to patient and back; anticipating the next horrendous round.

Moments in the Death of a Flesh Mechanic...a healer's rebirth

"How long to the hospital?" he asked.

"About fifteen minutes," I replied, checking my watch.

"That means we can look forward..."

Ben was cut off by a gurgling sound from the patient, followed by an immediate response from the radio.

"Medic Eight," Dr. Gilroy said, "it looks like your patient just went into fib again. Confirm. If so, defibrillate at 200 joules."

"Affirmative, Dr. G.," I answered and then dropped the radio transceiver to charge the paddles.

Ben, familiar with the routine by now, gave the patient a couple of quick breaths with the positive pressure mask and then positioned himself over the patient. I was ready, so I motioned him aside and put the paddles on the patient's chest.

Mr. McArthur opened his eyes and looked straight into mine. He opened his mouth to talk at the exact second I hit the buttons and discharged 200 joules of electricity into his chest, stopping his heart.

With an, "OHH!" his body hopped, his eyes shut. He fell silent.

"Was that a normal beat I just saw before you defibrillated, Medic Eight?" the doctor asked.

I fumbled for the radio and dropped the handset. Compressions were renewed. *Ben was working on someone I just killed!* All I could see was the man's eyes looking into mine as I extinguished his spark!

I purposely shifted my attention to Ben to distract myself. I didn't want to answer the doctor. Ben was doing compressions with his whole body, his whole heart, his whole soul. At first, his eyes were fixed on the cabinet in front of him, but as he put all he had into the task, he began looking down at a space somewhere above the man's chest.

"Status, Medic 8?" asked the doctor over the radio.

Ben's lips were moving. I knew what he was doing. He was imploring, ordering and cajoling the man's life spirit to choose life. As if in confirmation, at the peak of each compression, instead of calling out "One, and, two, and, three" like you do when maintaining a steady rhythm, instead he called out; "Don't...crap...out...dammit...DON'T!"

Now, there were *three* people in crisis in the back of Medic 8 as it streaked toward Santa Maria at 90 MPH! I picked up the handset.

"I...I put him out." was my ragged, delayed reply to the doctor.

"Hit him again," the doc said.

As I did what I was told, I swore under my breath that never again would I use the word "hit" to describe cardiac defibrillation!

We waited for what seemed forever for the flat line produced by the shock to snap into a heartbeat. Mr. McArthur, on his own, took in a breath and then opened his eyes again. They were bloodshot, but alive. He rolled them up toward the ceiling as if to say, "What a trip!" and then closed them again.

Ben and I both turned away from the patient. Ben twisted his leg toward the door leading to the front of the unit and stared out towards the road, now intersecting with Highway 101, the last stretch to the hospital. His leg was shaking uncontrollably. I repositioned the monitor so I could watch it and the stark side wall at the same time.

As we turned away, however, each of us put out an arm to put a hand on the man. Our hands touched for a second and then followed through until they landed on opposite shoulders of the patient.

"Medic 8," asked the doctor over the radio, "ETA and status?"

"We're about three minutes out," I replied; "Please be ready!"

Mr. McArthur made it to the hospital. Within a few minutes, he was rolled to the Cardiac Care Unit. One minute after that, he went into cardiac arrest. This time, the doctor decided to intubate and start a central venous IV line on him. Prior to that, intubation had not been an option because the man might have tried to pull it out during times of consciousness. By now, Mr. McArthur, too, was beyond exhaustion.

Over the course of the next hour, our patient went into and out of cardiac arrest another five times. Luckily, he never regained consciousness. His veins absorbed just about every drug in the book in combinations that were probably never attempted before as two cardiologists, an anesthesiologist and a surgeon made a valiant effort to help him to stay on this side of the line.

Whenever CPR had to be done, either Ben or I was there to do it. If Mr. McArthur were to be one of the very lucky few, we wanted to be a part of it. Or maybe it was more because we needed to make him alive to apologize for the torture we had just put him through.

Once again, as it had many times in my career, the thought of quitting this patient — hell, the whole biz — danced through my head. I'll never win. Not really. But I wasn't ready to give up my role, either, which was to be the advocate as best I could, a consistent presence in the battle until the scales tipped one way or the other, as if to remind God that He created us in His image.

Ben was doing compressions when, after 15 minutes of asystole — flat line, *no* heartbeat — the doctor said, "Okay...we're through now."

Moments in the Death of a Flesh Mechanic...a healer's rebirth

Ben kept his hands on Mr. McArthur's chest, discolored blue and red from multiple electric shocks and compressions. As I had done so many times before, I knew he was feeling for whatever was there.

The emptiness in Ben's expression died as he lifted his hands off the man and looked at them for what seemed a long, long time. He wiped them on the stretcher's sheet and then stepped off the stool he was standing on to provide leverage for his compressions.

He walked out of the cubicle, looking for some reason for it all. I had no answers to help him; all I could see was Mr. McArthur's eyes.

We both sat with Mrs. McArthur a few minutes, just after she was given the word that her husband had died. She had been spared witnessing any of his last moments.

"Just two minutes ago," Mrs. McArthur said, "it seemed as if this would never end; like it would go on forever. The waiting; the not knowing; now, it seems like it was all over so fast."

She turned to Ben: "It did happen very quickly, didn't it?"

He took the woman's hand and grasped it thankfully. Then, he looked around the room as if trying to be absolutely sure where he was. He looked directly into her eyes and with both a reassuring and reassured smile on his face, and unafraid of letting a tear show, he answered:

"Yes, it did."

Chapter Thirteen

TEACHING TERESA

"Here," I said, "let me show you."

I leaned over the ambulance stretcher and gingerly took the woman's right forearm in my hands. I took care not to disturb the IV in it, or her left arm, which was snugly wrapped in bandages. The sleeve of her loose cotton pajama top, soaked pink from watered-down blood from the bathtub that she had been pulled out of a few minutes earlier, was already rolled up above her elbow.

"Next time," I continued, "pull the telephone cord out of the wall, or cut it, or just unplug it, for God sakes. Then, it won't matter if the phone gets knocked off the hook. And, if you're serious, take the razor blade and slice *down* the veins, not across them."

As I drew an imaginary line with my finger from the bend of her elbow down to her wrist, she looked on raptly, appreciatively.

"That's harder for the doctor to repair," I explained. "Bleeding is more profuse. The wound is less likely to seal itself off; it's faster"

I spoke evenly, as if it were a one-on-one in-service session. The middle-aged woman, Teresa was her name, nodded her head.

"I haven't seemed to be able to do anything right or very well, have I?" she asked me evenly.

Not quite true, Teresa, I thought, you seem to be on schedule. I wasn't quite sure what that meant, either. For some strange reason I was appreciative of this moment with her. It certainly hadn't started that way.

As soon as the call had come in over the radio, I started cursing to myself. I knew the address, I knew who it was, I knew what to expect, and I even knew what the conclusion would be — a couple months from now, the same thing would repeat.

By the time I went into the house, I had let whatever compassion I had in my bones drain out. On this call, my intention was to *be* a Flesh Mechanic.

Moments in the Death of a Flesh Mechanic...a healer's rebirth

This was the third time this year I had been part of this woman's sad story, and all three of them starred suicide...attempted suicide, excuse me. The truth is, I was sick of attempted suicides, successful suicides, threatened suicides; I was sick of them all.

She was lying in her tub, weak but alert. Her brother, shaken, and with this odd, furtive look on his face I thought, was holding her left arm up and putting pressure with both hands on a huge wad of toilet paper, dripping with blood. The straight razor blade she had used was still sitting on the rim of the tub.

I moved swiftly and professionally, watching and listening to her breathing, noticing the color of her lips, checking consciousness, examining the wound, wrapping it, handing her arm to her brother, checking vitals, starting the IV and, then, with my EMT partner, lifting her on the gurney and out into the back of the rig. I was looking forward to getting away from people. I wanted to be alone with her.

As soon as the doors were closed to the passenger compartment, I started in on her while I set her up with some oxygen.

"Teresa," I said quietly but with an edge, "this is getting old."

"Sorry to inconvenience you." she replied, not angrily or apologetically, but factually, as if cutting through a crowd and nudging me aside. Something about the way she said it prompted me to look more closely. Times in the past I had been with her she was defensive.

"It's not about me, and you know it." I said. "I told you the last time. Some day, someone's gonna die who wants to live 'cause I'm screwing around with you. You have any idea how inconvenient *that* is?"

I was busying myself cleaning up the drug box and speaking to her in a conversational tone. I feared if I started to let the charge I was feeling squeeze out, the dam would burst.

Serendipity is a reality to the medic. It had caused me to be dispatched to almost wherever Teresa had been when she made a new attempt at taking her life. During the last couple of years, I also happened to have participated in a string of deaths of vital people who so much wanted to live.

I found myself treating a pre-teen boy with heart cancer; a girl whose first motorcycle ride with her boyfriend resulted in being hit broadside by a van; a young man on military leave that broke his neck; and an older artist who was in the midst of finishing his masterpiece when he was struck down with a heart attack. They were so unlike most of the other critical patients I had come across.

In each case, these people were struggling with everything they had to stay alive; fighting so hard for something as simple as the next breath. Every one died. Until their last second, each fought valiantly.

What does that look like?

Sometimes, breathing ceases. But it doesn't just cease. The last exhalation is complete and total as if the breath of life itself leaves every cell. Now and again, you can literally see the animating spirit of the being leave as well. There is a perceptible change in color, something you can see, but it's elusive as the "Green Flash" at sunset over the sea.

That's where the "death rattle" comes from. To the uninitiated, it's an exhalation that never ends! When you hear it, you know it's a flat line; the heart is gone. Of course, you get the bag-mask ready, knowing there's no hope. But before you can get the mask over her face, the patient suddenly takes in a tortuous breath as if she were starving for air, which, in fact, she was.

For a minute, both of you thought she was dead!

Other times, you first see it in the monitor. The electrical activity in the heart peters out. Then, the body loses any semblance of tension and lets go. Sometimes the bowels let go as well. Then, even before you can begin CPR, or see increased activity on the monitor, the body tenses again. Then you notice an effectual rhythm working itself on to the screen, as if being willed to come forth.

The only reason I use the above examples is because they are rare instances. They are rare because they can be described. The more common experience would be the medic "sensing" the waves of struggle and release; struggle and release. Sometimes, even with vital signs still present and clinically sound, you know that particular struggle is over. But if you feel anything at all — and granted at times it's 90% your own hopes — you work for it.

Hopes? Of course there are hopes. The whole purpose of the job is to bring back the dead if you can. If there were no hope, why would anyone bother? I think medics of all stripes forget that part of the emotional fuel that drove them into the profession in the first place was the chance to play a part in offering that very hope to those who, not too long ago were once the hopeless.

As my patients struggled to keep their lives, I fancied myself battling as well. When events turned in their disfavor, I worked that much harder because I believed I had connected with their desire to live. At times I could feel life leaving their bodies and the core of their life force struggling to bring it back and hold on to it. Other times it felt like something out "there" was reaching in to take the life inside for itself.

The harder my patients struggled, the more I invested, somehow trying to match their soul's efforts with mine. It may very well have been a total fantasy on my part that I was actually fighting *with* them. But does it matter? To intercede takes energy and commitment. It has to come from somewhere and can as easily come from an emotional connection as it does from a sense of professional pride and duty.

Moments in the Death of a Flesh Mechanic...a healer's rebirth

As one struggling death heaped upon the other, however, my own weariness multiplied. By my fourth exposure, for days after I was drained: What my hands felt in those crucial moments broke my heart.

Of course, I had to pick myself up and find reason to move along with my own life. *But then I'd be called upon to deal with people who were young and healthy and wanted to throw it all away?*

For the most part, it was a dance, a game, an act-as-if for me, a place where, like an actor in a bad play, I had my lines and my role, and that's what I delivered; *Flesh Mechanic par Excellence* you might say.

This wasn't the first time I had told an attempted suicide I'd prefer to be helping someone live who wanted to. It didn't happen often, and only with repeats, but still, it was inevitable given the number of such calls I had to run. Too many ambulance calls are about providing a chance to live to people intent on seeking death!

It used to be I wanted to pass on some sense of responsibility to them, to inject them with the idea they actually *do* affect people. What I said never really had an effect; they were wrapped up in themselves, I decided, so I stopped trying to be the one to re-instill their will to live.

Teresa didn't feel wrapped up in herself today. Not like in the past. Today, there was a quality of resignation in her I hadn't noticed before; and something else, a sort of strength.

Something was brewing in me, as well. It dawned on me, loath as I was to admit it; I had a relationship with this woman. My life had intersected with hers at very crucial junctures. I knew this woman at her most human points, and something had changed in her. I was a little chilled by it. But I couldn't help myself; I wanted to know more.

I stopped my busywork and just looked at her. Her eyes were staring at a space just above her feet. It wasn't a vacant stare; it was more a look of solid determination.

"What are you doing?" I asked, "Where are you at?"

"Thinking."

Whenever she ended up in my ambulance, whether I liked it or not, I got another glimpse into her life. Her distaste for life hadn't seemed honest to me. There had always been an edge of her playing, toying with the idea of ending it. It felt more like she wanted to run from her life, which is different from wanting to end it.

I'd do my job; get her to the hospital alive. I'd even lecture or question her. The last time, I yelled at her. She, like so many others, was a drain; on everyone in her life, the system, me, and *your* pocketbook. I couldn't respect her because she really wasn't serious. That makes it feel like we're all being jerked around for fun. But today, I sensed something was a bit different.

"Let's face it, kiddo," I said, maybe wanting to test her, "you must not have been completely ready to check out today. Neither were you ready the last two times before that. How many other times did you try when it wasn't me that picked you up this year?"

"Two others."

"Five times this year!" I exclaimed, "What's that tell you?"

"I'm incompetent?" She asked seriously.

Most people I pick up screw up the attempt once. The second time they figure it out and do it right; if they're serious. Either that or they quit and just get on with living as best they can. I wasn't trying to shame her. My point was valid. People who are really intent on suicide commit suicide. Quietly. Irrevocably. If ever there's a bit of wavering, a doubt, often it won't be successful.

True, there are accidents, where, in a "call for help" they just happen to get the technique right and do themselves in. To decide what is a call for help gone awry and what was the genuine article is a crapshoot when it comes to drug overdoses and flesh wounds. The ones who are intent, however, leave little doubt, for their choice of vehicle is irreversible. Most often, if not dramatically throwing themselves in front of a train, or well-planned hangings, it involves guns. It's the ones who are serious that I was comparing her to this day.

One day in Florida my partner and I arrived on a scene just prior to the Sheriff. We had both been dispatched to check out the concerns of a panicky family member who had received a "disturbing" phone call from her nephew, across town.

The relatively small house, on a corner of a typical residential neighborhood, had a thick wall of tall bamboo encircling it. Me and my partner cautiously knocked on the locked door, and getting no answer, walked around the side of the house to the back yard. We passed through a corridor of bamboo and both stopped in our tracks, awestruck at the sight of the garden.

Apparently, it was an Oriental garden of such design that it radiated "peace" as soon as we entered it. Not knowing anything of Feng-Shui at the time, I was bowled over by the precise, evocative beauty of its design. My partner was no less stunned. I literally felt a wave of peace, contentment and serenity wash over me. It was an incredibly long moment, but only a moment because it was part of our steady approach to the back of the house.

There was a walkway that went between the rear door of the house and a free-standing garage beside it. When we looked into the open garage we saw a body hanging from a rafter, a thick rope tied into a perfect Hangman's Noose around his neck. His face was bulging blue — clearly dead. Closer examination showed the man had stepped up on a rickety step stool, slung the rope around his neck and then shot himself in the heart with a small caliber pistol. This Dude *was* serious!

Moments in the Death of a Flesh Mechanic...a healer's rebirth

"I've tried pills...twice." Teresa said, "I even tried gassing myself. What more can I do?" She wasn't pleading. She was asking a direct question.

"The phone keeps getting in your way for one," I replied. "It did this time for sure. You left it off the hook, and your brother got alarmed. You knew damn well that he doesn't stay away for very long at a stretch. He leaves the house and you think about it and you think about it until maybe just an hour before he comes home, you decide to do something. But by then, he's home and we get called. To be honest, Teresa, your tactics and timing suck."

My response was measured, factual; even with concern. Teresa and I *did* have history. She made half-assed attempts to do herself in, and I ended up intervening. But I didn't have the luxury to be half-assed about saving her.

"And then, look what you did; Valium! The first time I picked you up, you OD'd on Valium. And that was your second try with pills, too, remember?"

Teresa looked around the interior of the ambulance trying to avoid my steady gaze. Then she abruptly turned and challenged me.

"Yes, but I did take twice as many the second time, the time with you."

"Maybe booze would have helped." I went on, annoyed this time. "Valium just takes too damn long to work. Somebody's bound to find you. Didn't you get that from the first time?"

"I worked with what I had, for Chrissakes!" She glared at me.

"Okay, Teresa." I smiled at her and softened. I couldn't help but chuckle at this absurdity.

I kept my eyes fixed on hers as I talked. She raised her head and, for the first time in our history, met my gaze. In her eyes I could see her spark and it had a certain quality — a kind of distance to it. I had seen this before in others' eyes, and it chilled me. The first dead body I had attended to had the same look in her eyes in the week just before she willed herself to death. Something deep inside was going away. But I wanted to be absolutely sure.

"And then the bit with the car. First of all, you're supposed to run a hose directly from the exhaust pipe into the cab of the car. Don't just sit in the garage with the car windows open; it takes too long. There's more of an opportunity for someone to find you."

I wasn't chiding her. I was just recounting our experiences together. There was a twisted intimacy about it.

"Don't get me wrong," I elaborated; "that should have worked. But what the hell possessed you to hold onto the garage door opener?"

I couldn't help it; I smiled at how I was getting as ridiculous as the whole scene. To my surprise, so did Teresa. We must have both pictured the same image, for she began to laugh.

"It was *habit*, Russ," she explained, "After I started the car, I went back into the house to feed the cat and brought the opener in with me. When I came out, I grabbed it like I always do. I didn't even realize I had it in my hand when I got back in the car."

And when she passed out, she tripped the button, the door opened; a passerby saw the car idling away in the open garage and called the police. The cops pulled her out, and we revived her.

"When I got to your house that time...and today, too," I began, for some reason suddenly curious, "I was more worried about your brother. Christ, Teresa, you're driving the poor guy nuts! What's the deal with that?"

"If I don't live with him, I'm homeless," She looked down to the floor. "He molested me when we were young...for a long, long time."

"Oh." That stopped me in my tracks.

She had nothing to hide. Whether I liked it or not, I got another glimpse into her life to add to the picture pieces I had picked up the last two times I had been with her. They didn't add up. None of the pieces of a life that leads one to suicide really add up for those who choose to continue living.

The first time I picked her up, during her second overdose, she was distraught after having had a visit with her daughter, who had been taken away from her 12 years earlier. Teresa had been diving into cocaine at the time, and her live-in boyfriend and she took off for a weekend, leaving her six-year-old girl alone in the house. She was taken out by a fireman responding to the fire that resulted from her trying to cook a frozen meal on the gas stovetop. Her hands had been burned.

Teresa had tried to regain custody, but ongoing drug problems and instability over nine years pretty much closed those doors. Teresa straightened up about three years ago, and waited until her daughter turned 18 to approach her again. The first day I met her was that day. Her daughter had just told Teresa she'd visit her again — at her funeral.

To her credit, Teresa somehow kept her head above water and stayed away from drugs. She found a new boyfriend in the church she attended about a year before I met her. Unfortunately, he was physically abusing her. He was killed in a terrible car wreck after they'd been living together for six months, just after the incident with her daughter. He was not alone in the car. She followed this up with two more attempts.

Teresa broke her eye contact with me, dropped her smile and stared out the back window with a look not of exhaustion, but a deep, deep tiredness. It was the same sort of tiredness you see in the beaten-down elderly, but with an edge. There was no doubt in my mind now. I was sure the shift had occurred. I was probably the only person in her world who could recognize it.

Whereas all the other times I had been with her she had a helpless pall about her, now an expression of otherworldliness had come over her — as if she had already gone. That had been the tip-off for me. The times I had picked her up before, she had a look on her emotion-beaten face that was a perpetual "Why me?" Now there was that peaceful look of surety. Why didn't matter any more. The switch had turned on and I sensed an Oriental garden nearby.

The majority of people who flirt with suicide stay in the limbo of not wanting to be *here*, but they are not quite willing to do what it takes to get *there*. How many of us choose the slow route? It is a true commitment to suffering. When the switch is tripped, however, there is a drive, not so much for self-destruction as for the person's experience of everything to cease. Her weariness was genuine.

It came to me I owed her the truth. I sensed until a short time ago she didn't even really believe suicide was something that was real. All that had changed. I wasn't sure when it had happened. It may have been after her last attempt. It may have been right there in front of me!

To be less than honest with her would have been disrespectful of the very human process she was going through. It was my duty to make it real for her. Not because the harsh reality might change her mind, but because without the knowledge of how it works, she could never make an appropriate choice.

And choice is so sacred, even God doesn't fuck with it.

Or perhaps it was because I sensed she really didn't understand what "final" looked like. All of this I knew in my heart. It was not in my thinking. So in that moment, I resigned myself to discuss things I had never discussed with another human being under any circumstances.

When a big rule is to be broken, breaking a few small rules along the way makes it seem justifiable. Just before I started my lesson, I breached professional etiquette and posed Teresa a challenge.

"You're ready," I said, "aren't you?"

"Yes," she replied without a moment's hesitation and looking me right in the eyes. It was then I knew; the choice had been made. For that is what suicide is all about; Choice; right or wrong.

There was a part of me that wanted to kill her, yes. Not for her, but for me — to get her out of the way from taking me away from my real work, which was to help people live who wanted to live. I was still very raw from my losses.

At the same time, I knew the role I had truly chosen was to participate in the struggle, no matter what it looked like; that's what I had signed up for. If everyone faded away peaceably, I'd have no job. This was a struggle. If there was life here somewhere, it was my job to find it.

As time had gone on in my career, I found myself feeling a respect for the people who did do suicide right the first time — those who successfully pulled their own plugs. They interpreted their lives, decided to act on that interpretation, and then did it. They didn't burden the living by holding them hostage as witnesses to their years of agonizing until they made up their mind.

What they did was make a final statement, one that left the rest of us to wonder "Why?" The most disturbing question wasn't why they choose to die. The question was why do *we* choose to continue to live?

For me, who was called to many cases like this, that question cropped up time and time again. So many of my calls were about futility, senselessness, and hopelessness; how could I not find pockets of my own life reflected there? Besides, everybody's headed for death and 99.9999% of us will die in obscurity without having budged the world an inch. Very few of us will *not* be completely forgotten in a few hundred years!

Each and every time I dealt with a suicide call, I was left with the afterglow of questioning my own desire and will to live. I was reminded that living is indeed a choice.

One of the pet illusions that helped me to justify my role in the struggle was the belief my actions were buying time for my critical patients so they could make the choice to either stay or go. As if, in the glow of that otherworldly light, they would confer with God and out of that come to clarity from which they could both make a better decision for everyone.

When someone moves to take his own life, however, it seems he is trying to usurp the will of God. Of course, that is absurd. The will of God is what happens. Suicide is a thing that happens. It, too, must be the will of God.

How could I second guess that? My job was to do whatever I could to preserve life, and I suppose it's *regardless*.

But when someone has truly crossed the line into being serious about killing himself, nothing is going to stop it. I saw that pattern repeat itself time and time again. We see people like this every day among us; it's just a matter of time before death catches up to the desire. To the paramedic who deals with the most extreme of these cases, after enough exposure, it's not too difficult to spot the ones who've made the decision.

I first saw this when I was fifteen years old. A friend of mine from High School's Dad had a collection of Classic cars. Every now and again, he'd steal one and take friends on joyrides. Over a year's time, the rides became more and more reckless. Something in his eyes started to change, but it was more violent than what I saw with Teresa, yet, like her, something was moving away. One day, with five of us in a Mercedes, he played Chickee with a School Bus.

I stopped riding with him. He was hell bent on something I didn't want to be near. One day I got stuck for a lift and ended up riding in the back of his Willy's Jeep. Riding right in the middle of a narrow country two lane road, we rounded a turn and smacked head-on into a 15 ton Bell Telephone truck! It was my only accident with injuries (a dislocated shoulder). No one else was hurt. Two years later he died in a high-speed motorcycle wreck. Alone, thank God!

For the more gently suicidal, before the switch is tripped attention is spent on re-living details. It appears like relentless self-absorption. After, it becomes a fixation on the act. I've been on car wrecks where recognizing one of the drivers, I was sure it was an attempt and last minute chicken out, but there was no way to prove it. I knew Teresa would not rest until she had completed the act.

The restlessness in her was so potent, and the part of her that had already left was so big, I found myself wanting to see her in peace even if it meant death. At rest; for that was the only place I knew she could come to oneness. But I was a paramedic, and I still had a job to do.

"I've changed, Russ," she said as I checked her bandages for the spread of blood. Her wound had stopped bleeding.

"I know. I'm sorry."

There were no more pretenses. No more lies.

"Oh," she said, "It's not bad, you know."

And then, she said factually, without fervor but filled with conviction: "I know now," she concluded, "there's nothing I could do to myself that would be more painful than staying alive."

Her words sent a chill up my spine. I had to counteract it. "Still, you keep botching up, Teresa. What does that tell you?" I asked.

Maybe I shouldn't let her get away with it, I thought. I half expected her to follow my lead and say something like "Maybe I want to live?" but she didn't. I still held to the belief I could make a difference.

She turned to me again. Looking me straight in the eye, she asked, "How then? What have I been doing wrong? *How do I do it right? Tell me.*"

At first tensing every muscle in my body, I wanted to run. When I first formed the idea of discussing such things with her, it seemed so straightforward; I'd just give her a lesson. But being in that moment now, everything changed.

How sure was I? How arrogant about claiming to know where she was at? But then I wondered; how many others had heard her ask questions they were afraid of and denied them with a "Don't be silly."

I felt compelled to oblige her and honor her by speaking the truth. So for the first and the last time in my career, I discussed with a patient how to do herself in, and I didn't stop at describing one method.

About two months after my partner and I had dropped her off at the hospital, I ran into her brother at a shopping center. At first, I didn't recognize him as he motioned to me, but then the memory clicked. He came up to me.

"You know," he said, "I never got to thank you for the kindness with which you treated Teresa."

His words surprised me, given what Teresa mentioned about the relationship. I chose to take a real good look at him. Just a guy, I thought, and accepted his gratitude, thankful to be thanked by anybody for anything. I remembered the last moments I spent with her and inside I winced.

"How is she?" I asked.

"You hadn't heard?" Without waiting for my reply, he told me. "A few weeks ago, after she had been doing rather well, actually, she started taking long hikes. One day, she packed up a day pack with food and then followed old San Marcos Pass up to Highway 154. She kept walking until she got to the Cold Springs Arch Bridge..."

I knew what was coming. I vividly pictured the bridge in my mind. One of the few metal arch bridges remaining in the country, it spans a divide between two mountains. To the south of it are green rolling mountain tops; to its north, a breathtaking view of the Santa Ynez River Valley and then in the distance, the Sierra Madre Mountains. Ahead is Lake Cachuma. It is a truly wondrous spot. Free. Unfettered. Expansive. About 150 feet below it, there is a rocky terrain of boulders, hard earth, and scraggly, thorny mesquite and scrub oak.

As he said the words, "She walked to the midpoint of the bridge and jumped," I pictured her smiling and hopping over the rail.

"Someone saw her," he said. "As he drove his car across the bridge, she was just standing there. Then she turned toward him and climbed onto the rail and leaned over."

I was relieved that the last act of her life, "flying" in ambulance parlance, was something Teresa had thought up all by herself.

Chapter Fourteen
LAST WORDS

We're following a smoky wind devil of dirt and dust and debris as it skips across a Tombstone Territory-like town's gritty Main Street. We hear a gunshot, and the wind devil loses power and dissolves. In the space it left behind, we see two men, 15 feet from each other in the center of the street. One stands, smoking gun drawn. The other sits on his behind, staring in semi-wonderment at a red stain spreading steadily across his shirt under his badge. His right hand spasms over the wound.

Hangman, the black leather-clad victor, cockily puts his gun back into its holster. He spits thick brown phlegm and tobacco juice on the ground and takes a satisfied look at the dying man. He turns and walks to his horse.

One of the saloon whores is the only citizen with the guts to go to the aid of the terribly wounded man. She flutters to him, dress billowing in the oppressively hot wind. Three members of Hangman's gang, astride their horses, automatically cock the hammers on their handguns and make ready to fire upon her. Hangman, mounting his horse beside his thugs, motions them to relax.

The sheriff could care less about the gang. He looks up at the whore imploringly. His glazed eyes reveal he's sinking fast. She moves behind him and helps him prop himself up so he can lean back on her.

"I guess..." The Sheriff starts to speak, but a cough rips through his body. He gags and then grimaces. A line of frothy, bright red blood rolls down the corner of his mouth.

"Just lay quiet now," she says; "someone's gettin' Doc."

The whore speaks gently as she nervously looks around. Save the cutthroat gang, she and the sheriff are alone on the street.

The sheriff makes a wracking cough. Blood sprays from his mouth in a fine mist. The Hangman chuckles and starts to move his horse forward to lead his gang toward the Sierra Nevada, looming above the town like tombstones. The sheriff opens his mouth again to talk. He clutches his chest over the bullet hole tightly. He summons from his depths the last bit of strength he has, and, as we come in closer to his face, whispers to the whore.

" Fitchville..." He takes in a deep, wheezing breath and holds it a second, and then says, "Henry...Parson." Some bloody spittle runs over his bottom lip as he pushes the words out of his mouth.

The whore strokes his head as if he were her child. She doesn't notice her dress dripping with blood from the bullet's exit wound. She listens intently.

The Hangman lets his horse amble up alongside of the dying sheriff. He pauses and leans over to hear:

"...I'm (weaker now, his hand drops to his side)... his...Fff..."

The sheriff lets out a wet, resigned sigh.

The Hangman sits up in his saddle and motions his men to pass.

The sheriff's head goes limp and flops back on the woman's bosom. Shaking, she eases herself back until his body slumps to the ground. Terror turns to horror as she looks down to see the blood all over her dress. Thrusting her hands to her mouth, she shrieks!

The Hangman looks at the woman with something resembling concern. "It's O.K., Ma'am." He says, I'll be goin' through those parts later. I'll be sure the boy gets word."

The Hangman mockingly tips his hat at the whore and grunts out a great belly laugh as he turns his horse around and then jabs his spurs into it, galloping away to catch up to his cohorts.

Most of us get to hear last words through speakers hidden near flickering screens. In the safety of the dark, we watch television and movies as images of the dying appear. They pull the last spark of energy left in them and form it into words that say it all and then, life is over. Sometimes, that spark gets stretched into a soliloquy!

Last words have something to do with the assailant, the higher-up, or the crime, often forced out of the dying person by one of the living. The speaker knows something everyone else needs to know. Last words are essential, for without them, the *plot* would die!

At times, the words cleanly sum up the life of the dying person: and start us on a journey, like "Rosebud!" They may be a wry comment that floors us with tragedy and truth, like, "should've turned left."

How those words affect us, and that's just on the screen! To actually play witness to them; to be there and hear the key-tap of the final period in the story of a life is a sacred experience; something indelibly etched into one's memory like the day you lose your virginity.

Moments in the Death of a Flesh Mechanic...a healer's rebirth

How can we not wonder what our own last words will be and who will be there to hear them? There are so many good ones out there! Perhaps ours will last as well.

Doesn't it seem strange to you that so many poets, writers, artists, entrepreneurs, statesmen of prominence, or people with some form of notoriety, got to get off such perfect exit lines? Take Karl Marx, for example. These are his last words of record: "Go on, get out! Last words are for fools who haven't said enough!" Perfect — and succinct, and, well, powerfully lively!

The speakers seem to have hammered out their life's philosophy into a few well placed phrases, uttered them, and then checked out with the same presence of mind as if they had been ordering wine and cheese at their local Bistro.

In ages past, it was common practice to have someone in attendance at the bedside of the great and mighty for the express purpose of recording those last thoughts. Obviously, after the fact, there was picking and choosing going on.

In doing a cursory search, I found many of the most popular quotations showing different stories from different sources, or what appeared to be contrivance in a desire to leave a lasting legacy. Bottom line, I thought to myself, "Yeah, Right!"

The popular impression as expressed in media is the last breath is at the heels of the last words. The final comment offered by John Sedgwick, speaking of his troops' vulnerability during the battle of Spotsylvania Courthouse in the Civil War, illustrates this. Witnesses reported he said, "Why, they couldn't hit an elephant at this dist—"

In reality, those are true last words, and they are extremely rare.

Having been a part of a few hundred deaths over my career — deaths where my first contact was while the spark was still glowing with relative strength — I have been amazed at just how few cogent last words have come to my ears, and almost none accompanied by the last breath.

The human body is a phenomenal machine; built to protect itself on many levels. When it comes to the final battle, the body is quick to eliminate rational thought, the least of ingredients central to the fight. The last thing to show up in our evolution is the first thing to leave!

Unconsciousness or delirium set in and the dying are spared the burden of accurately perceiving and experiencing the event. The initial shock of trauma provides a psychic numbness, attributable to the overwhelming number of injured cells screaming out for attention; like trying to recognize one voice amidst a sea of yelling fans in a stadium.

The psychic and physical energy needed to overcome the Grim Reaper is too valuable to waste on words; or even screams! I realized this while watching the classic movie *Jaws*. There was Quint, being chomped by the teeth of the shark as he is being sucked into its belly; screaming like a loon! Do you think for one second in the real world, he would have had the spare energy to scream the way he did? People who come back report they were distant from the worst part of their "dying" experience, and believe me, Mr. Quint was quite preoccupied!

Usually, the time surrounding the moment of death appears peaceful. The person lies seemingly uninvolved and uncaring; if there is any fight, it plays out subtly, perhaps in a twitch. Only in the rarest of circumstances are there visible signs of struggle. It is most often something sensed, not seen. When the very few *do* struggle for their lives; it's devastating. When you experience it, it rocks your world. But for the most part, death is personal and something that is not shared.

As a qualifier, my experience does not include war. Movies I've seen or books I've read portray the agony and struggle soldiers go through in battle. It is a noisy and ugly and public thing and soldiers are screaming and gasping out last words left and right. I've never been to war, mostly only personal, little wars, so I have no frame of reference. All I can share is my experience in the civilian world.

I attended a Pre-Hospital Emergency Medicine conference in Florida once where the Chief of Detectives of the Miami Police Department gave a presentation on principles for the management of a crime scene by emergency personnel prior to the arrival of the police. His lecture consisted of simple yet important tips: Take mental notes on the physical set-up of the crime scene; take care to disturb as little physical evidence as possible; and render efficient and unobtrusive care to the victim. He concluded by saying the only thing left to do was to listen carefully to anything the victim would say. "Especially the last words..." he said, "...write them down if you can." and then he laughed one of those laughs that are laughed by one who knows better.

I had no reason to question him at the time. I was a relative newcomer; eyes agape with wonder and the will and desire to take in everything at once. It wasn't until many years later I recalled his laugh.

It was in the back of an ambulance during a balls-to-the-wall ride to an Emergency Room in Santa Maria. A boy was dying and everything in me said it wasn't fair. Worst of all, I shouldn't have even been there; I should have been on my way home. I wished I had had the stamina at the time to follow through on my regular routine.

I had been commuting to work from San Marcos Pass to Orcutt, a town on the outskirts of Santa Maria, by motorcycle, a trip of some 50 or more miles. Riding home after being relieved of duty at 8:00 a.m. was an unpleasant prospect that morning. A blanket of Santa Maria-style fog lingered and made the air thick, biting and chilling to the bone.

Moments in the Death of a Flesh Mechanic...a healer's rebirth

After my partner left and I relinquished control of the unit to the oncoming crew — Matt, a paramedic, and Fred, a young, rookie EMT — I tried to stave off the inevitable. I talked to the crew, took a real long shower, made breakfast, talked to the crew, sat and read, talked to the crew, waited and waited for the fog to burn off; anything but to get on that damn bike!

Obstinately, the fog persisted. Time passed; the emergency bell clanged and, rather than face the prospect of sitting in that volunteer fire station alone forever, I slipped on my jumpsuit and hopped into the unit with the new crew.

It was no big deal. Medics are used to their cohorts suddenly riding along just for the fun of it. Each of us knows normal life, for the most part, can be pretty boring and see no reason to begrudge the other a little action.

This call had all the trappings of being a good one; an emergency call of an unknown nature from one of the oil leases in the foothills. It could be anything, and certainly offered enough promise to put off wrapping my legs around that cold steel machine and facing my teeth into the thick wet wind.

Sitting on the jump seat in the rear of the unit, I raised the head of the gurney to a sitting position and hooked my feet around its frame and braced myself for the trip. The ambulance flew through town in a flash; there wasn't a whole lot to Orcutt.

I watched as houses planted in cow pastures on the east side suddenly gave way to long fields furrowed with brown rows of earth awaiting seed. A few short hills and then a series of new fields surrounded with carefully aligned fencing around them. In these fields were boney grape vines appearing like arthritic hands hung in rows waiting for the healing warmth of the sun.

The ambulance, siren wailing, rumbled up and down a set of hills and broke through the fog into bright and cheery sunlight. Cresting another hill brought the fields we had just passed into view. I pictured them flushed with bright green leaves and grapes. The sunlight warmed my legs and I savored it.

Once over a higher set of hills, the land lost its order. Fences were more traumatized and less aligned. The land's surface was rough and barren, and uneven. Gray streaks of road starting behind thick metal gates ducked between hills and seemed to go nowhere. Metal signs tacked on fence posts announced strips of land leased by a slew of oil companies: a strip for Chevron; a strip for Union; a strip for Texaco...on and on through the bare hills.

A man stood at an opened gate and motioned us in. Sliding into the dirt roadway, we passed him as he urgently motioned down the road. We must have traveled for a mile when, reaching the top of a sharp hill, we had an overview of a long valley with a row of eleven huge oil derricks. They looked like a colony of rigid grasshoppers, pounding their heads arrhythmically on to the ground.

The road snaked down into the valley and the ambulance made a bee-line for one of the pumps with a conglomeration of people, cars, and trucks gathered around it. The closer we got the heavier the syncopated rhythm of the oil pumps' *CA-CHUGGA, CA-CHUGGA* vibrated through the ambulance.

There are advantages to riding along on an emergency call and not being a member of the primary crew; the pressure is off. Unless it is some sort of multiple/multiple victim situation, a two-man crew can handle whatever comes up. When it is a one-patient call, a rider can usually have the luxury of observing, getting the feel of the call, and filling in with a lot of supportive actions and information that allows the crew to function more smoothly.

The payoff for the ride-along is in not having to experience the tension that comes with carrying the major responsibility. There's comfort in being able to play a role helping make everything run like clockwork. The third man is available as back-up, and usually available on the request of the primary crew. That's the theory.

On this day, I was an observer. I didn't have to be there. Soon the fog would burn off in the valley proper, and I knew I would be on my way home. I casually stepped out of the ambulance after the main crew and noticed them quickly move to a figure collapsed in a heap on the ground. I walked up to a gaggle of oil workers who had left the side of their co-worker to make way for the medics. They were pale and shaken.

"I jus' cain't…the damned fool knowed better." A burly man with weathered skin and brick hands shook his head and yelled over the *CA-CHUGGA CA-CHUGGA* of the pump before I could ask anything.

"I couldn't even find whar the bleedin' was comin' from, there was SO much," he continued. I noticed he was shaking.

I looked down and saw a foot-wide swath of blood running downhill from the collapsed man's leg. I heard Matt bark out orders to his rookie to get a tassel of equipment.

"He jes walked into it!" The worker said.

"Walked into what?" I asked as I looked down and now could see that one of the man's legs was grotesquely mangled and laying attached to his hip by no more than just a few strands of flesh — essentially an amputation.

"The fuckin' counterweight! What th'hell else you think could whup a man like thet!" He pointed angrily at a thick anvil shaped metal block as large as a shopping cart basket. It whipped around in a circle, balancing out the steady up and down motion of the long pump arm supporting what could be called the "head" of the grasshopper. He looked at me like I was a dumb shit.

With a steady backbeat of *CA-CHUGGA, CA-CHUGGA, CA-CHUGGA* lending a surreal aspect to the scene, for a moment, I felt as if popped into the middle of some metaphoric science fiction story. The mammoth metal grasshopper, intent on its chore, relentlessly sucks fluid from the earth. Meanwhile, an innocent man, pledged to assist the creature, lay broken and bloody beside it, his own precious fluid replenishing that which has been taken.

Something caught my ear: The medics were in trouble. They were so intent on what they were doing they stopped talking to each other. The silence was the tip-off. They hadn't spoken to each other for too long. I drew closer to get involved and see if I could help.

Fred was searching for a good place to apply pressure on the man's leg to stave off the steady but now slow loss of blood. He was having no luck, not with direct pressure over the uppermost part of the wound or with pressure on the man's femoral artery. The wound was close to the hip. An improvised tourniquet was ineffective. There wasn't enough room on the man's leg to secure it above the extensive damage.

Matt was making his third attempt to start an intravenous line in the man's arm, to no avail. In the first crucial moments after his leg had been struck, he must have lost enough blood to collapse his veins. This, coupled with his muscular arms and tough, skin, made it almost impossible to place a needle.

I rushed to the unit to get the M.A.S.T. suit. Matt, in the meantime, had made the decision to spend no more time on the scene and to get the man to the hospital as quickly as possible. In the most serious of cases, which this was, the only therapy and the best judgment would be to load and go. The best the paramedic program had to offer could only waste precious seconds getting the patient to the hospital where more ideal conditions and expert help existed.

I quickly helped Matt and Fred wrap the M.A.S.T. suit around the man, scoop him, inflate the trousers, and put him on to the gurney and into the unit. Fred got behind the wheel. Matt managed to get an 18 gauge IV needle in place in his right forearm and began running fluids. At least it was something. Then, he got in contact with the hospital to warn them to get ready for us.

At first, outside at the foot of the gurney, I used pillows to support his leg, raised the foot of the scoop to put him into Trendelenberg anti-shock position and helped him free his arms so he could put them across his chest. I then got in to the ambulance and sat on the small jump seat above his head, and leaned over him, while Matt worked on him from the side of the gurney.

The persistent and annoying *CA-CHUGGA, CA-CHUGGA* faded in the distance. I chose to stick with the patient and make him as comfortable and stable as possible — back to the basics. I knew it would be a long, hard haul.

He was a boy no more than 19. He had been alert, conscious, and slipping. By now his vital organs were seriously depleted of oxygen and nutrients. Distant, his words came softly, like out of a haze.

"Am I bad?" The voice spoke, but his eyes did not meet mine.

"Not too bad," I answered, somewhat automatically. I knew fully well he had bled out right before my eyes.

This was not how I wanted things to be, how I wanted *me* to be. I didn't know where this was leading, but I felt drawn to just be with the kid, to answer his questions. It must have been the child in both of us.

A pause of, to me, an interminable amount of time — perhaps two full minutes — occurred. The ambulance careened through the back roads of Santa Maria while Matt, leaning over from the squad bench at his side, made another attempt at an IV on his left arm. The boy/man looked up at me for reassurance. I reached down and grasped his right shoulder and stroked his head gently.

Matt was unsuccessful. By now, he was shaking. He turned to the radio again. I decided it was time for me to intercede and take a crack at an IV. I reached forward to palpate the boys left arm for a good vein and the boy grabbed my hand and held it startlingly tight.

"I'm not gonna...?" His words trailed off. I felt him shiver. His skin was getting colder to the touch. He loosened his grip.

I could not let go.

Drawing in closer to him, as close as I could in the rocking ambulance, I continued stroking his head. No answer came from my mouth because, now, I had none. He drifted into unconsciousness again, and I was relieved.

Perhaps in those moments, I noticed where the previous attempts at an IV had been made, and where there was still room to try; the external jugular, for example. And I may have noticed whether or not the oxygen flow was high or low, or if the pressure in the M.A.S.T. trousers was holding steady, but something kept me in my role. I was bonded to the patient, but more important, to the moment, and in this moment I had no doubt, I was with someone who was dying and nothing me or anyone else could do would change that.

Then I started screaming to myself. I wanted to retreat into the safety of "treatment." My mind said it was bad for me and bad for the patient for me just to sit there. The face of the only patient I held myself responsible for killing flitted past my mind's eye. "For Chrissakes, you're a fuckin' paramedic. DO somethin'!!" The words screamed in my head.

I looked down to see the patient had become a boy to me; just a frightened boy who was dying. He shuddered again and this time he opened his eyes. He looked up toward me. I prayed his eyes wouldn't meet mine in part because I knew the last thing *he'd* see would be someone dying; a Flesh Mechanic entrusted with saving his life.

But our eyes did meet. I drew my head down and closer to his so I could meet his gaze because it was his eyes that sought mine out. All I knew was I was exactly where I was supposed to be; spending an eternity with this dying boy.

Moments in the Death of a Flesh Mechanic...a healer's rebirth

I felt tears sliding down my cheeks but it was okay. I felt strong because they were there to wish him well on his journey. He was simply a pioneer in whose steps I'd soon be following. I was at peace with that.

I stared into infinity while Matt crawled around me, tending to this, adjusting that, calling in the other; filling his world with superstitious behavior in the belief it could stop death.

I watched the boy's spark recede into the distance of his eyes. I realized *Something* was going somewhere else That's what I was watching! Something was going somewhere else. Maybe I was just on the other end of a birth. Could it be that *these* were the births of which I was meant to be part?

And then I shuddered at what I noticed next; *my face in his pupil*! He was no longer a victim, nor my patient; he was my reflection.

Mercifully, he shifted his gaze downward. Smacking his lips, he said — unconcerned and as a statement of fact — "Cold."

I held his hand the remaining two minutes to the hospital. The boy looked asleep, but I knew he was somewhere else. I let go, and got out of the rig to help Matt take the gurney out. Before we made it into the Emergency Room, the boy's heart stopped beating.

I noticed the fog was as thick as when I had awakened that morning. I dreaded the cold ride home like I have never dreaded a ride before or since.

Epilogue

We were dispatched Code Three to a nursing home in Santa Barbara. We went careening into the lobby, gurney laden with our equipment, expecting to be met by a nurse. There was no one to greet us, of course, nor was there a sense of urgency in the air.

We walked up to a central hallway, where we had a choice of three corridors to follow. Not knowing where to go, and realizing life was peaceful in the hallway and it wouldn't make sense to cause a commotion, we stopped dead in our tracks.

I asked Patrick, our ride-along, to go to the nurses' station down the hall and find out where we were going.

Patrick was an Explorer Scout. He was about 17 and had ridden along with me and many of my partners religiously for the past two years. The program was designed to have Boy Scouts go out into the real world with firemen, policemen and medics to earn skill badges that moved them into higher and higher levels of the Scouts.

When he started, he was just a hot-dog kid, in love with lights and sirens. Over the years, however, I got to watch him grow into a young man who truly enjoyed the work and the people, and he was conscientious as could be. I worked with him for an up to eight-hour shift perhaps once every three or four months, so I got to see how he used whatever he was taught from other medics.

I enjoyed teaching him the basics because I didn't have to stick with any sort of guidelines. I could teach him how to think like a medic, and that's exactly what he was learning to do.

That year, around my twelfth year in EMS, I had my grandest political victory. From day one, I had been struggling to get paramedics the support and recognition they deserved; one battle after another. If it wasn't with the company, it was the county, or fire department, or the police department, or even local doctors and nurses. In those earliest years, there were even confrontations with undertakers!

Moments in the Death of a Flesh Mechanic…a healer's rebirth

Private ambulance companies were notorious for having poorly maintained vehicles, inadequate equipment, and miserable hours, pay and benefits. Counties went with the lowest bidder on a contract; you were never sure for whom you'd be working the next year. Whatever you were offered in pay and benefits, you had to take.

I got adept in communications. I'd articulate the workers' positions and then present it to the company or county and meet with committees of my fellow workers. I learned how to get free publicity to force the public's attention to issues at hand. I learned how to organize.

Every company I worked for considered me a rabble-rouser. I had the personality defect of calling things as me and my peers saw them. When it came to improving services made available to the people, it was the medics who had to lead the charge. The system just wanted things to be open for business and really didn't care too much about how well the service functioned (unless it garnered bad press!), or how those who provided the service were looked after, or how often they burned out.

My involvement went in cycles. A new challenge would come up, like the county accepting a bid from a company that wanted to increase hours and lower pay for the medics. I'd find myself investing energy and hours upon hours doing whatever I needed to do to rally the medics, get a position, present that position to whoever would listen, including media, and then lobby, lobby, lobby. After all failed or was successful, I'd crash and swear I'd never get involved in politics again!

For three years, I was involved with a number of committees and associations. They were focused on making people more aware of paramedic services, lobbying for improved equipment and county-wide standards, and bringing the pay, benefits and hours of county paramedics to a level commensurate with other vital agencies.

At the time, in 1985, our pay and hour differential was at least 25 percent below city and county fire department personnel. That last year, I was working a mandated fifty-six hour work week, at top level of pay for the company based on experience, and making $5.60 an hour.

Every time we came close to having an agreement, the company would scuttle it, back down, or begin and then renege on the deal. Even though I was a New Yorker, where I grew up hearing, "Unions screwed everything up!" I began to listen to one of my partners and we decided to seek a union out to represent us in negotiations with the company.

As Communications Officer for the movement, whose core included five other co-workers, I handled anything that went out in print to the medics, the company, the union or the press. I scheduled presentations and took polls and educated county medics on the history of failed relations with the company and county, and this very new vision of gaining professional representation for our concerns.

How the company hated me! It was not a pretty campaign. After about a year of six of us medics investing tons of our own time and money, working with lawyers and officials, raising money and doing everything by the book (okay, almost!), it went to a vote. Over 80 percent of the medics in the company voted in an affiliation with a union, part of the Service Employees International Union (AFL-CIO).

I lobbied long and hard to include a clause that I created. The contract drawn up between the California Paramedics Association and the union stipulated that we would be represented in bargaining agreements only, while we retained control over how we pursued anything that had to do with promoting paramedic services.

By not being part of the union but affiliated with it we were able to assure that we would not be obligated to strike if that were deemed necessary to further the progress of other Locals of the union. The union would provide clout and experience for provider negotiations; period. Our ethical obligation, first and foremost, was to the patient.

This was unprecedented. The CPA was not a union for EMS workers; it was a professional association with union affiliation. At the time, unions were struggling to regain a foothold after having spent years getting decimated by Ronald Reagan's policies. Remember the Air Traffic Controller's Union's strike because conditions were making it almost impossible to do their jobs? Our President stepped in and fired every one of the strikers!

Just a short time after having been part of the team that may have revolutionized EMS (but didn't); I was trying to find a patient in a nursing home once again!

Patrick pointed to his left, and Dave and I started down the hall to the end of the corridor and its nurses' station. The nurse on duty, unconcerned about anything as usual, handed me a chart.

"'B' bed, room 118," she said.

"We got called in Code Three," Dave said.

"Well, that was a mistake!" the nurse said with a smile. "She's a slow GI bleeder with a stable blood pressure. We can't do any more with her as far as her stroke goes. She just needs to get to the hospital."

Of course, we didn't trust her.

The three of us went into the room to find an 80-year-old woman, conscious but not very with it, and in no apparent distress.

Dave had Patrick check her vital signs, while he hooked her up to the monitor ("May as well, we dragged it in here!"), and I looked over the chart to see what kind of blood pressures she had over the last few days. Everything checked out. Indeed, this was a non-emergency.

Moments in the Death of a Flesh Mechanic...a healer's rebirth

Calling in to the dispatcher to find out why she had called it as a Code Three, we found she based it on the RN saying the patient was a GI bleeder; emphasis on the word "bleed". We explained the situation and told her we'd be going Code One, a non-emergency transport.

The woman had been in the home for a month. She had no fewer than five grocery bags of belongings, two big boxes, and three poinsettia plants. Our job, since we were professional paramedics, was to load her and all she owned into the back of the rig and calmly drive a few miles to her new home.

We all carried her stuff and rolled her out to the ambulance bay. Patrick got into the unit from the rear and positioned himself at the head of the gurney while Dave and I collapsed it and handed the patient in to him. Then, we started to hand in the bags. One by one, they took up all the extra space in the back, and Patrick was essentially, though not inextricably, wedged in to his corner of the ambulance.

Now, what? Dave and I discussed it. Both of us felt confident in Patrick's ability to do basic monitoring. We told him to keep monitoring her all the way to the hospital, 10 minutes away, and let us know if there was any change whatsoever. Any sliding downhill that the woman had gone through in the last month had been slowly incremental. There was no reason to suspect there would be a sudden turn now.

We each felt comfortable with leaving Patrick in the back of the ambulance. I drove, and Dave rode shotgun. If anything were to happen under any circumstances, we'd all have to mobilize and throw all that shit out of the back of the ambulance to make space to work her up anyway!

We pulled out and went a few blocks. Naturally, there was our company's shift supervisor, sitting in his ambulance on move up. He saw us both in the cab, and knowing we were transporting a patient, followed us to the hospital.

After getting the woman situated, we explained what happened to the supervisor, William. We had a chuckle; another bizarre ambulance story! William mentioned we were the crew he could most rely on. Even though unionizing had expanded the rift between management (paramedics themselves, like William) and employees, we could count on William to work with what he experienced, rather than anyone's agenda.

"Given the climate of things around here," he said, "I need to go by the book and fill out an incident report. I'm going to recommend a written warning to be put in your files." No big deal. It was fine with us.

Wow, did the company go to town on that one!

Two days later, we were fired. Then, our State Ambulance Driver's Certificates were revoked. Then, our Santa Barbara County paramedic certifications were pulled, and, for good measure, our unemployment insurance was denied! They claimed we were guilty of "gross incompetence in the performance of (our) duty." In one fell swoop, my career in EMS, professional reputation, standing in my community, and ability to get employed in my chosen field were ruined!

I spent the next nine months in hearings, interviews, and reviews all over Southern California. My record as a medic was picked apart. In some hearings, my partner and I were considered together. I filed an Unfair Labor Practices complaint with the National Labor Relations Board. The union worked with me on my defense in front of the NLRB, but I was on my own with all the others.

One by one, I had all certificates and licenses and benefits completely restored (1986). There was no evidence of incompetence as claimed. It was a judgment call, and under the circumstances maybe not too sharp, but within reasonable limits in terms of patient safety.

I did not ask to be reinstated, nor did I want to apply anywhere else. It was time. The politics did me in, not the work; I was burned out.

The NLRB ruled against my claim the firing was in retaliation for my prominent pro-union activity. With an almost prior spotless record of my own and the company's history of only firing two other people in the last five years for infractions that far eclipsed my own, the conclusion seemed almost unfathomable.

The union did not, in my opinion, defend me aggressively in that Reagan-era, reactionary hearing. Once the verdict came in, I never heard from them again. I suspect I was the sacrificial lamb. Now, I guessed, it was the Union who didn't need a rabble-rouser on board!

I filed a lawsuit against the company, giving $1,500 to the lawyer who was supposed to be the hottest guy for this stuff in the state. He was a boozehound who dropped everything he was working on, including me, as his life quickly unraveled. He got disbarred and filed bankruptcy on the money I had given him as retainer.

My partner during those last glorious days of my ambulance work used the momentum from his being fired to propel him into law school. Eventually, he filed a lawsuit against the ambulance company — representing himself (not me!) as part of his curricula. He won!

As for me? I kept following the moments, one after another, making sense of my experience and applying that knowledge to the healing arts until I ended up right here, in your life. *Thanks for making the trip so very worthwhile!*

www.ingramcontent.com/pod-product-compliance
Lightning Source LLC
LaVergne TN
LVHW051557070426
835507LV00021B/2623